NUTRITIONAL ALIGNMENT®

HELENA COLLINS

Nutritional Alignment © 2012 Helena Collins.

ISBN:978-0-9886602-1-2

Published by Life in Synergy Press

Written by Helena Collins

Edited by Meghan Kavanaugh

Cover Image by John Forcucci

DEDICATION

I love the words thank you

Here are some of the most important ones that I need to share.

To my husband Brian, the light of my life and the most amazing person I have ever met.

To the thousands that have come up to me and said, "Can I ask you a question?" that inspired me to write out some answers.

To Meghan Kavanaugh and Ilana Katz, my editors that taught me how write and then, edit, edit, edit.

To Marissa King and Susan Holtzman, many thanks for your honest input and support.

To my entire team at Life in Synergy®:

Alexis, Candace, Charlie, Chrissy, Emily, Grace, Heather, Jenny, Jessica, Joanna, JoEllen, Lauren, Samantha and Shay, thank you for helping me spread the Life in Synergy spark to the rest of the world!

Finally to Ryan Deiss and Perry Belcher, thank you for helping me understand the process of getting this book to the public.

Helena

Table of Contents

Spread Good Karma

If you like this book, spread the good Karma!

Leave us a review on Amazon, We would truly appreciate it!

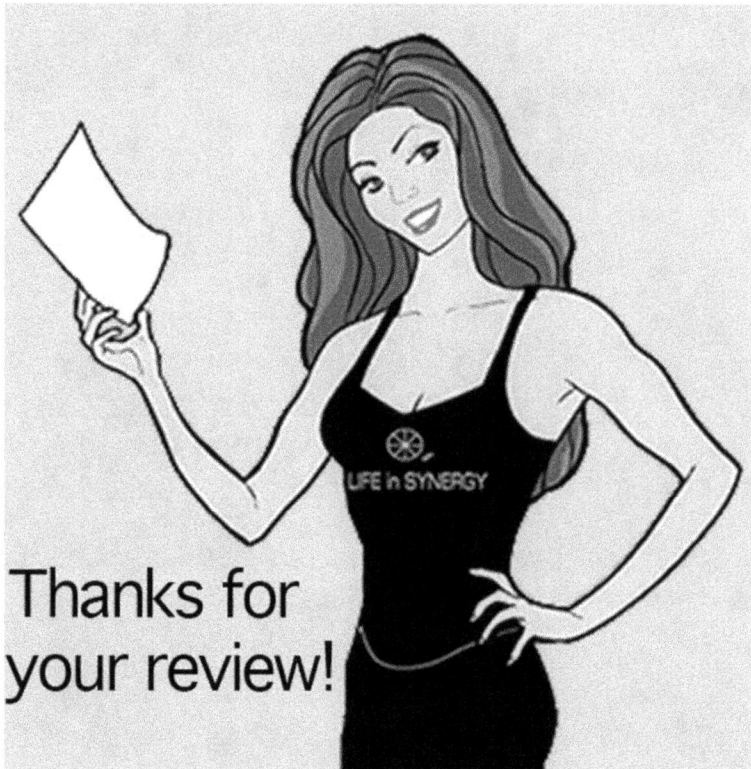

Thanks for your review!

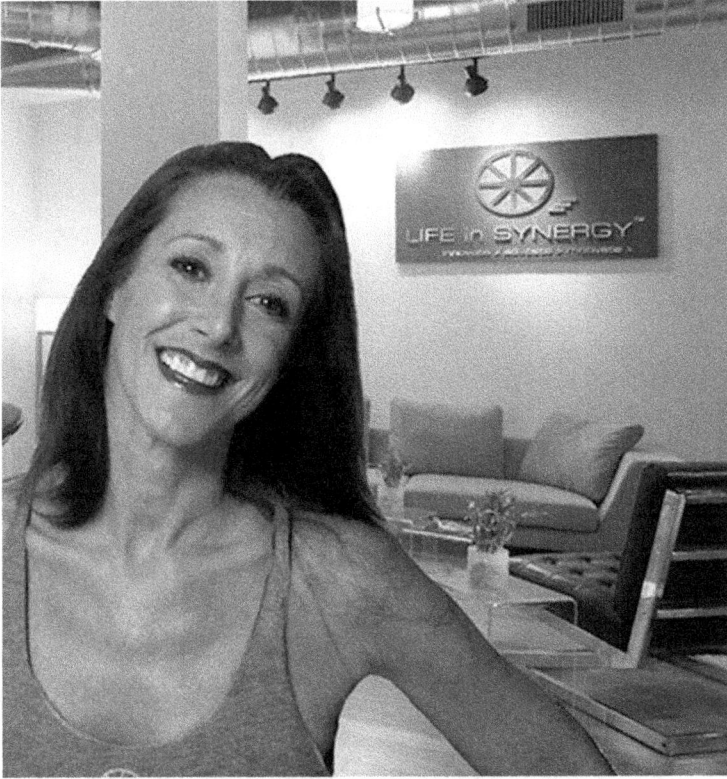

About the Author:

Helena Collins is known as the Hott Maker.

The founder of Life in Synergy® as well as the developer of the Synergistics Fitness Method®, Nutritional Alignment®, Walking and Water® and Mind in Synergy programs. She is a multi-award winning personal trainer, teacher and wellness consultant for individuals and corporations and has helped thousands around the world live at their ideal weight and transform their lives and their bodies.

Her career, spanning over three decades has included intensive cross-cultural Synergistic study of varied mediums and practices, such as meditation, spirituality, pilates, yoga, martial arts, chi-gong, tai chi, chinese medical theory and the traditional sciences of physiology, psychology and nutrition.

Introduction to a Life in Synergy with...
Nutritional Alignment

Here is an e-mail I received recently... I cannot wait to receive a similar one from you:

"I loved Nutritional Alignment. I have lost 15 lbs.! I completely reworked how I saw food and weight loss. Before I lost weight, I never realized how much of my day was consumed with me feeling bad about my body. Now that I know my number and know how to eat, I actually feel like I have MORE freedom to eat what I want and not feel guilty.

Thank you! I am ready to be free!"

Are YOU ready to be free?

Helena Collins

Don't Diet, Align!

Whenever you hear, "Everything in Moderation", do you just want to get up and throw something at the TV?

What does that even mean? And of course, this kind of statement usually follows a cooking segment on a morning show that has just taught you how to make the most Divine double chocolate brownies and precedes a recommendation from the latest diet guru or nutritionist to eliminate carrots from your diet because they have too much sugar and have a high glycemic index.

High protein, low protein, high carb, low carb, glycemic index, cleanse, fast, prepackaged cardboard food, ugh! The whole thing is exhausting.

Are you searching for a way to live more fully and enjoy life, to be at the weight that feels best for you physically and emotionally without having to starve or beat yourself up? Do you want to LIVE, to stop worrying all the time about every bite of food you have or don't have? If you are ready to stop dieting, if you just want to LIVE, then Nutritional Alignment® is for you.

The journey behind the discovery

Twenty five years ago, I was managing a gym, writing training manuals for instructors, weight training, and leading aerobics classes. As one of the very first certified personal trainers in the country, I was a rising star and leader in the fitness industry, presenting at numerous national workshops for instructors.

Despite my growing success, there was something seriously wrong. I was never happy with my body. I was constantly forcing myself in to workouts I did not enjoy, suffering from chronic back and knee pain, starving myself and still, I could never get thin enough to like my thighs. I knew that there had to be a better way.

A way to love my body, my thighs and my life. A better way to teach the students that I genuinely cared about, other than to tell them to do more and eat less. I knew to my core that as a born teacher (I taught my first students violin lessons and swimming lessons starting at the age of 10) that I had a responsibility to not only teach but to inspire my students to LOVE what they were learning.

With a belief and a desire for real answers and real possibility I pursued a path towards achieving this "better way" and found myself on a personal journey that would ultimately change the lives of thousands of women. Over the next ten years, it demanded a learning trajectory that spanned intensive studies of cross-culture mediums and practices.

I spent countless years and hours studying pilates, yoga, martial arts, chi-gong, tai chi, meditation, spirituality, chinese medical theory and the traditional sciences of physiology, psychology and nutrition. Yes, you guessed it, I am a full-blown geek. (Really, I was a Mathlete in high school.) Each time I studied these new disciplines I would totally immerse myself in them so I could not only excel but also fully understand what changes and benefits each discipline would have on my body and my life.

It was through the scientific process of testing, analyzing and re-testing that all aspects of my Life in Synergy waterwheel were born.

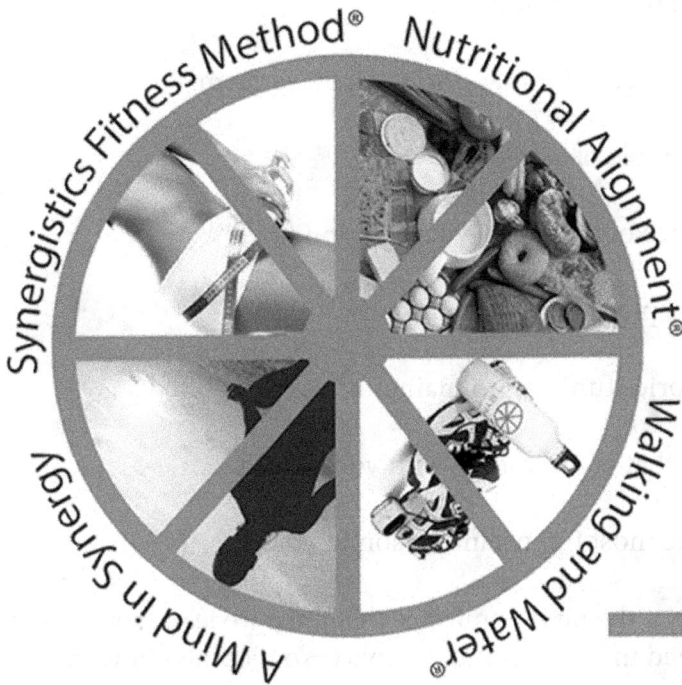

This segment of the wheel, Nutritional Alignment, often has such a profound impact on the women I teach that I knew it deserved to be the first book in the Life in Synergy series. Nutritional Alignment is the combination of all of these sciences and disciplines I have studied to make it optimally effective.

Eating is not just about nutrition.

It is:

•Feeding your emotional, mental and physical bodies

- Understanding how your subconscious mind takes over and why you find yourself eating out of habit or stress

- Understanding your taste buds and why you have them

- Understanding the role of gender

- Learning the science of nutrients, vitamins and fiber

- Understanding the physiology of your body

- Learning how calories function to maintain mass

- Creating your life that is in Synergy with your world

- Learning about the most important person in your life, YOU!

The great thing about the human mind is that once we learn something, it becomes engrained in our every day activity. You learned how to brush your teeth and put on mascara, now you are going to learn how to eat to be your ideal weight for the rest of your life.

Once you learn it, you will be done forever!

A multi award winner decides to write a book

My name is Helena Collins and I live in Boston, where they call me the "Hottmaker".

I have a reputation for making smart women hott. We will get in to the full definition of hottness in a minute, it is not just about being thin or fit. It is about being happy and fulfilled and enjoying life, all the while having the body of your dreams. Smart women, you are my group. The women in the world that are ready to look at diet and fitness in a whole new way. Smart women have questions and are looking for answers that satisfy them. Smart women want to know the how and the why! Sure, I work with some brilliant men who are ready to learn, but mostly, it is women that flock to me in search of a solution that does not involve a 1,000 calorie a day diet or 5 days a week in the gym.

Over the past 15 years, I have been here in Boston, teaching and personal training. First with my multi-award winning personal training studio, Synergistics that I opened in 1997. But I was always thinking about all of the other people to reach and teach. In 2008, I opened Life in Synergy, where I have been able to reach more people eager to learn. With the addition of classroom space in my new larger studio, I began teaching this aspect of the wheel, Nutritional Alignment as a seminar, I could not offer that class often enough. It would sell out in minutes every time, with women flying into Boston to join their friends and family to learn! Still not satisfied with my ability to reach all those desiring to learn, I turned the seminar in to a 30-day online class that has reached women all over the world. Still, there was so much more I had to say and the idea for this book was born.

While the awards and accolades I have earned over the years are amazing and really appreciated, the real thrill for me as teacher is in the success of my students. Every time that I receive an email like the one above, there is added happiness in my world, and the joy of knowing that there is another person out there that has truly been set free; no longer thinking or worrying about diet and fitness all of the time.

The true measure of my success is the success of others. I want you to be successful and send me emails :-) As you learn Nutritional Alignment and embrace your own Life in Synergy, you will have more free time in your day to create, to laugh, to love (especially yourself), and really live. I am excited by the contribution that each of you will be adding to the world! Imagine what you will do with your newfound energy, focus and valuable hours.

Let me be abundantly clear, I am not a physician or a registered nutritionist, so following the advice of your medical professional that knows your body the best is always the right move but, there is a reason that my studio is filled with Doctors, Physical Therapists, Research Scientists, Ph.D.'s and women from every profession that approach their jobs from an intellectual standpoint, from moms to make-up artists.

There is a method to working smart instead of hard.

I have discovered it, and I am excited to share it with you.

To share the the skills I learned to live fully, freely, and hott is an honor and a privilege, thank you for taking the time to learn about the most important person in your life...... YOU!

Read on to start living your own Life in Synergy!

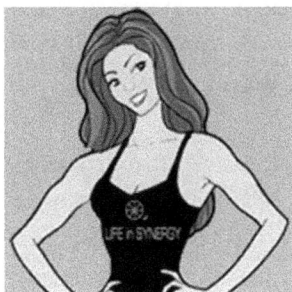

CHAPTER 1

YOU ARE NOT A LIZARD

Have you ever wondered why most animals are not overweight but so many humans are? What do they know that we don't? Why does food and eating seem so much simpler for them?

There is a reason.

Oh, the life of a lizard. One day you are born, popping out of your shell and your whole life is laid out in front of you. You will live in a nest near the river, you will drink water, you will eat flies, you will find a mate and have baby lizards. You will be on the lookout for snakes when your baby lizards are incubating and you will bask in the sun. End of story. This is the case for most of the animal life on planet Earth, but not for us.

The reason? Adaptability. To what do we have to adapt? Well, climate for starters, because humans are the only living beings on the planet that live in every climactic zone. We live on the equator and above the Arctic Circle, on the water and on top of mountains, in deserts and rain forests, and in cities and suburbs. Survival in each of these environments has different requirements. In order to thrive we need to understand our environment, learn about it and adapt.

Unlike the lizard, we are born without any pre-programmed knowledge. But the ultimate tool, our brain, is capable of learning, adapting and thriving in all of these different places. This is the part of your body that I am interested in, your brain. Your brain, your survival tool, is ready to learn whatever it needs to help you thrive in your environment. I do not know about you, but my environment includes cupcakes and wine. I live just outside of Boston. In my world, there are restaurants and barbecues and life. This is where we need to learn to survive and thrive!

The Life in Synergy Difference

Everything begins in our brain and everything we know we have learned.

This includes the foods you crave, the size that you have taught your body to be and the joy or pain that you feel each and every day when you look in the mirror or get on the scale. I want you to imagine getting up in the morning free from the anxiety about getting dressed, free of the judgment of yourself – not because you have learned to compromise but because you have learned to be in control and to live your life fully.

This is the Life in Synergy difference.

The Ultimate You

Instead of forcing you into another way of managing your life and your expectations, I am going to teach you how to realize and discover the ultimate you. I'll teach you how to fully live at the weight that will make you jump out of bed every morning and love the person that you are.

I will teach you how to make decisions for the environment in which you live. I am not going to teach you how to diet. Diets do not work. They are short-term programs that force your body into unsustainable habits but they never teach you how to live in a healthy, manageable and sustainable way. Are you really never going to eat birthday cake ever again? It is time to learn a new way of life, and understand how the ultimate you lives every day with all kinds of choices. Stop cramming for a test and memorizing facts that you will soon forget! Learn about adapting to a whole new way of life and embracing it.

I am going to teach you how to use your brain to program a new way of being. You are capable of learning to be anybody that you want to be. (Well, almost. I can't make you five inches taller. Sorry!) But I can teach you the skills to be the person of your dreams. Oh, I could feel that eye roll from here, accompanied by the thought, "Yeah right, you are probably one of those naturally skinny girls who can eat anything or that only eats lettuce." In actuality, most of my family is overweight, my genetics predisposition is towards obesity, and I just enjoyed a scone for breakfast.

Yes, on some days there is lettuce in my life (in fact, lately I have been fairly obsessed with arugula) but life is not about lettuce or scones, life is about understanding and enjoying it all without stress or anxiety. Oh, I can feel it, here comes the next one, "Yeah, but you probably work out all the time." There is nothing fun or healthy about exercising all of the time. I do not condone over-exercising. I do a few targeted workouts a week to teach my brain better communication with my body, and 10,000 steps every day in cute shoes. I do not run or do cardio. (How would I maintain my lipstick color when running?) Now, if you love running, I am not saying that you have to stop.

I am saying that your workouts are a time for you to learn about yourself and enjoy your body. Do not do them because you are forcing yourself. Beating yourself up is not healthy; it is abuse. I am the size I am because I taught my body to be this size. I learned the amount of food my body needs to maintain my body weight. I learned to listen to my body telling me to stop eating because it was full. I had to learn all of these skills. They were not pre-programmed.

Once I made the decision to learn, my brain and body were excited to change. As I understood and developed a great relationship with myself, my body, my environment and food, my own Life in Synergy emerged. A Life in Synergy with a Nutritional Alignment program is a life of fun, happiness, success, joy, enjoyment and hottness. I love this word because it encompasses a total way of being.

Hottness is feeling:

•confident
•sexy
•capable
•secure
•amazing
•in control
•armed with the knowledge to shape who you want to be and what you want your life to look like

It is time to get off that treadmill – literally and figuratively. It is time to be done with the never-ending pattern of weight-loss followed by weight-gain followed by decreased self-esteem. Partaking in programs of starvation teaches your body that you need to starve. I cannot tell you how many women I have met (I will introduce some of them to you) that were stuck in a constant diet. They never learned healthy ways to eat and, instead, managed every bite of food.

Whether they were overweight or underweight, they suffered from the exact same self-esteem issues.

This program teaches you how to eat, how to live a full life and how to have your very own Life in Synergy!

Where did this program come from?

Like I mentioned in the intro, being the geek that I am, I stopped looking at all of this as an emotional topic and began looking at it as an intellectual one. Instead of constantly wondering why I was not like that girl who could eat anything and never gain weight, I analyzed the science behind maintaining human mass. I began to study and started with a list of questions.

How many calories does it take to maintain a certain-sized human being? Why is there such a variety of foods to choose from in the human diet when lizards only eat flies? What is the purpose of each food type? Why are there all of these different tastes, and why do I crave some more than others? Like a good researcher, I experimented first on myself and then with countless others, to come up with this program.

Remember, the part of your body that I am interested in is your brain! As you learn why you need different foods, why your taste buds crave certain foods and not others, why you might want a salad while your husband wants a steak, it will all become clear. Knowledge is power. Instead of just saying, "eat this," I am going to tell you why. You will be empowered with the understanding of how to make educated choices for yourself.

This new knowledge will improve your relationship with yourself. By the way, that girl who can eat whatever she wants?

In all probability she does not eat as much as you think, but even if she does, who cares?

Not me. The only person I care about right now is you.

I'm going to help you realize what a complete and awesome rock star you are.

Your most important relationship

Back to you. What does it mean that you need to improve your relationship with yourself?

Throughout your life, you will always be with yourself. This is the most important relationship that you have – you with you. Think about how many details you know about a celebrity or an athlete. Do you know that much detail about how to feed and care for your own body? Every time I work with a woman I ask her who the most important person in her life is and she will inevitably list off at least ten people before she even thinks about herself. I like to illustrate this with the inverted pyramid:

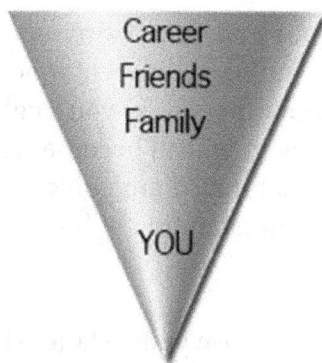

Career
Friends
Family

YOU

Think of all of the responsibility of having all of those relationships resting on the one little point at the bottom. The pyramid is a cone shape, constantly tipping from side to side, trying to hold up all of those people, problems, thoughts and jobs. No wonder we are all trying to instill some sort of management program in to our lives, or build ourselves up with extra food to handle these burdens. Unless you are completely still (and don't live your life to the fullest), living like this is impossible. The pyramid will fall and get a little beaten up.

You are the most important person in your life. WAIT! STOP! READ THAT AGAIN!

You are the most important person in your life. This is probably the hardest concept for women to learn. Throughout your entire life, you will change your style, your friends, even your beliefs, but you will never be able to get away from yourself. You will spend 24 hours a day, 7 days a week with you for your whole life. I know that this may seem obvious but it warrants pointing out.

Your relationship with you is the most important one you will ever have, and for women it can be the relationship most filled with strife. How often have you said, "I hate my ____"? Think about how difficult it is for you to say that about someone else, but how easy it is for us to say it about ourselves. We spend most of our lives trying to cope, and the remainder of our time thinking about the seemingly ideal lives of other people, and what they might be thinking about us.

Not only are we living with all of that pressure on one little point, but we are taking any extra energy that we have and spending it focused outside of ourselves worrying about the judgment that other people may pass on us. Whew! That was exhausting just writing it. Believe me, I understand.

I used to spend all of my time thinking about what other people where thinking about me, and I know that it does not leave a lot of time and energy to think positively about ourselves. First, let's flip the pyramid:

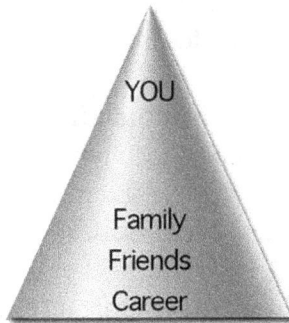

YOU

Family
Friends
Career

Now, you can see yourself on top. You are the CEO of your life. Think about the CEO of a major corporation. They are not spending all of their time at the whim of their employees, they use their time to effectively direct everything so that everyone can then do their own jobs more effectively and the team together can accomplish so much more than the individual. Not only that, but when you are on top you can better enjoy the people in your life.

I like to use the analogy of my ring. I love my engagement ring, every time I look at it, it makes me happy. But, if that ring was on top of my head, pushing down on my skull you can be pretty sure that I would not like it very long. It would hurt and be frustrating. I would be thinking, get that darn thing off my finger. This is what happens when we put others above us. Instead of being able to fully enjoy them, they become a burden, an annoyance, a problem. All of this has a ripple effect on everyone around us. It is the concept of self first. This is probably most difficult for my young moms to learn, though we all suffer from this either with our families, our jobs or our friends.

Self first does not mean selfish. You are the most important person in your life but you are not more important than other people. The way to look at this; does whatever you are doing improve your world while doing no harm to anyone else. I have a client Jane, she is an amazing Mom, but she was sacrificing herself for her kids constantly. This was leaving her frustrated and tired all of the time. Her Mom often volunteered to babysit but Jane was so concerned about what her kids where doing or eating that she had a hard time letting go.

She was in class one day when I was talking about this concept of self first and it was as if a light went off in her head. Her kids would be fine with her Mom for a few hours. The net result, they are all happier. Jane has a few hours to spend on herself. Her children are developing a better relationship with their Grandmother and her Mom is loving her time with her grandchildren. The important first step is that Jane had to embrace putting her self first. There are countless stories like this. I am of course not advocating that you abandon anyone, just that you make decisions based on what is going to add to your life and to the lives of those around you. (We will go in to more detail on this in one of the next books in the series, creating your Mind in Synergy.)

We have all heard "peace begins with me," so let's start. I will teach you how to be in control and at peace with yourself and your body. I did not say learn to compromise. I said be at peace, be thrilled with how awesome you are. Your relationship with yourself should be judgment-free and filled with love and respect. Think again about how often have you said, "I hate my _____"?

Think about how quickly you jump to criticize yourself and how these feelings then translate to how you interact with the rest of the world. Have you ever noticed how easy it is to snap at someone when you are frustrated about how your jeans feel? Or to put a damper on an exciting evening because you are unhappy with how your dress looks? It is time for these feelings to end and for your Life in Synergy to begin. Oh, I can hear the doubting thoughts start to surface now:

"But Helena, I wasn't born with super model genes." It does not matter. You where born with a brain that is capable of learning and adapting.

Once you learn something you know it for life and can share it with others. Stop the yelling and the torture, and start the learning and the loving. Sure, you're not a lizard, but you are an amazing, beautiful, capable human being.

Read on, and begin your own Life in Synergy journey!

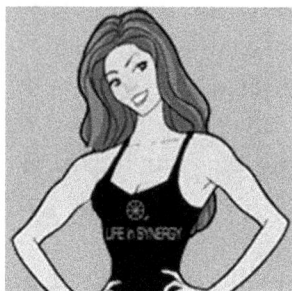

CHAPTER 2

YOUR BODY IS YOUR HOUSE OF BEING

In this chapter we will identify your dream house of being and then teach you the route to get there and move in for life. In order for a GPS to work you need to know where you are now, and to clearly understand your destination. Once you know these two key points, you plug them in and step-by-step directions appear. This is exactly how learning to navigate toward your Life in Synergy® and Nutritional Alignment® works. First you have to pick where it is that you want to live, and this begins by understanding where you are now.

This chapter: Explains the different elements of your body as your house of physical, physiological, mental and emotional health. Helps you assess the condition of your current house of being and how you feel about it. Walks you through the process of thinking about what your ideal house of being is. Don't hold back! It introduces you to the ways you can get the keys to unlock your ideal house and move in forever and make it a home that you love. It's not as complicated as you think!

Assessing your current house of being

Your body is your house:
Consider the elements of the house you live in and notice how this translates to the map of your body. Both are structures that depend on strengths of all kinds, and require knowledge to maintain them properly.

The Attic

Your attic is your brain, the important part of the house that keeps out the inclement weather, ventilates the hot air, and acts as shelter even if your house is just a lean-to. It is where you store your thoughts and emotions.

The Living room

The main part of your house, where you live day-to-day. This corresponds with the physical appearance of your body. It is also the part that you decorate and show off.

The Garage

Your garage is where all of the essential equipment that keeps your house functioning resides- the tool shed. This corresponds to your internal workings, the functional part of your body. These important parts of your house require certain fuel and maintenance to keep them working in top form.

Let's look at each aspect more in depth, recognizing that you may need to learn elements in each segment in order to ultimately maintain your ideal new house and turn it in to a home that you love forever.

The Attic:

Answer the following questions:

•Do you put the opinions, thoughts and needs of others before yourself?
•Does your body exhaust you?
•Does your body embarrass you?
•Do you feel like you must compromise because you could never afford or have an awesome body?
•Do you feel unable to keep up with maintenance so you think, "why bother trying anything at all?"

If you answered yes to most of these questions, you are probably a thinker.

The Thinker

The thinker needs to explore the attic section of their personal house of being. They have usually stored so much up there, both mentally and emotionally, that there is no room to move around, and no way for the hot air to escape to keep their house well-ventilated. The air in their home is trapped and not circulating.

Here is an example of classic thinker:
Sue is incredibly intelligent. She is well-informed and loves to research anything and everything about food, life and art. Her weight has been all over the map, from a size 4 to a size 24. She was always starting a new diet or coming up with a new way to manage her weight. Instead of her body being exhausted at the end of the day, it was her mind. She was not only constantly thinking about herself, but of what others thought about her.

There was just too much thinking. Instead of trusting her own roof and attic to keep her sheltered, and cover her in a storm, she was spending most of her day thinking that somebody else's house was better than her own. Instead of maintaining the shingles on her own roof, she was spending that energy looking at everybody else's, and then comparing herself to them. As she slumped home exhausted at the end of the day, she would reach for her comfort foods.

I asked her, "If you wake up tomorrow morning disliking the way your body looks, and feeling bad about yourself, were you really comforted by those foods?" I have to tell you, the look of realization on her face was amazing! Her ideal weight is an intellectual issue, not an emotional one. Now, before she eats anything that used to be deemed "comforting," she asks the important question – will eating this bring me peace today and tomorrow?

Once she realized that real comfort was not found in food, she was able to look for comfort elsewhere, in books, music, art and friendship (especially the friendship that she develops with herself). As far as her comfort foods go, once we calculated her daily 1,820 calorie requirement (you'll learn the formula soon), she was able to assess where to fit them in her life in a comforting way. Because she loves sweets, we made a plan for her to get 300 of her calories every day from something sweet. Even though her sweet craving is naturally changing, by taking the stress and judgment away from it, she was able to assess what her body really wanted. No guilt, no stress, no obsessive thinking. She has an organized plan.

So far, she has lost almost 50 pounds, but the important part is that she is learning how to live in her dream house already. She is learning how much fuel is required to maintain her house and turn it in to a home.

Thinker Exercise:

If you are a thinker, here is your daily homework. Remember, we are just teaching our brains a new skill, the skill of loving ourselves. I like to say these statements in the morning, as well as any time my thinking brain starts to take over. If you are a thinker, you may want to spend a few days right here.

I put these statements on my phone, on my computer, on sticky notes – anywhere and everywhere so that I can see them when I need a reminder.

•I am the most important person in my life.
•My happiness is worth my time.
•I am amazing.
•My life is not a compromise.
•I am worth the effort.

Use this list, and add your own thoughts. You are teaching your ever-thinking mind a new language.

The living room:

Answer the following questions:

•Are you obsessed with perfection?
•Do you plan your life around exercise?
•Do you micromanage everything that you eat?
•Are you frustrated because you work so hard and still not feel good about yourself ?

Yes? Then you are probably a decorator.

The Decorator

The decorator is constantly micromanaging. The minute that anything is out of place they need to fix it. They have the cleaner out for the glass table before the meal is even finished. This person needs to learn about the main part of their house, and how to live in it.

Here is a great example of a decorator:
Jill is a beautiful woman – tall, thin and striking. But when I met her, I could not see any of that. She was stressed out all of the time. There was no joy in her. She was unable to fully love and appreciate her fabulous body. She was constantly fixing it, working on it and rearranging everything. Every day she was stressing about her workouts, running miles upon miles so that she could eat and still maintain her body weight.

She was spending four hours in the gym some days in order to keep her appearance the way she thought it should be. She couldn't meet her friends because she had to work out. Just like in an overly decorated apartment, there was never a time for her to relax and enjoy the beauty, no time to put her feet up on the coffee table and watch a bad movie, no time for a casual stroll and a cookie. In the pursuit of perfection, she was constantly afraid and stressed, which was not fun for anyone, including herself, to be around. Her obsession had led her to unhealthy and dangerous habits that ultimately were not making her sexy and hott, just stressed.

We figured out her caloric intake for an active woman of her ideal weight – 1,625 calories – and she bought a $10 pedometer. Instead of working out for hours every day, she clips on her pedometer and walks throughout her day with a daily goal of 10,000 steps. This freed up hours in her day to enjoy and pursue other goals and interests. She ends up taking a 30-minute walk every day, and then just goes about her daily routine. She is not beating herself up anymore. And in doing this, she lost the last five pounds over which she always stressed. By not micro-managing, her body was able to let go. Instead of constantly trying to keep everything perfect, she learned how to fully live and relax.

Decorator exercise:

If you are a decorator, here is your homework. Remember, we are just teaching our brains a new skill, the skill of caring for ourselves instead of managing our body and our lives.

•Make a list of the things that you love about yourself and your body, remind yourself daily about them.
•Pick a workout that you love, maybe dancing in your kitchen (yes, this is exercise)
•Schedule a weekly fun outing.
•Indulge yourself, this does not have to be with food :-)
•Remind yourself "I am worth the effort."

Feel free to add to the list and post your list where you can remind your-self of your new journey. You are teaching your decorating mind a new language.

The Garage:

Answer the following questions:

•Do you have good days and bad days?

- Do you always begin your workout/diet plans on a Monday?
- Do you live for the weekends?
- Are you working really hard but your body never seems to change?
- Nodding your head? You are probably a commuter.

The Commuter

The commuter needs to learn about their garage, how to properly fuel and maintain their ideal home. Cara's goal was to weigh 115 pounds, sustained with 1,500 calories a day. This was her fuel requirement, but Cara was stuck in the commuter mode of good vs. bad days. Every Monday Cara's workout and diet life began. Monday through Thursday of every week, like a job, she was on a permanent diet, restricting herself to 1,000 calories a day (which only fuels a 77-pound active woman), paired with long cardio workouts and some weight training.

During the week, her body was living on a death march without enough fuel, but with bouts of intense work that could feel like torture. By the time Friday came along, Cara's body was primed for the oasis. What had she taught her body? Not only was she in starvation-mode Monday through Friday, but her body was working double-time. Your body does not know that you are working out, it only knows that you are asking it to complete a task, over and over and over again. As far as your body is concerned, whatever you are teaching it is for its survival, so it learns and adapts so that it can be successful, and prosper. Every week, Cara was teaching her body that it had to be beaten up, that it was going to starve.

Once Cara arrived at the weekend, her body shut down. Full-time couch and full-time eating. When we calculated her caloric intake on the weekend, she was eating to be a 300-pound woman (almost 4,000 calories a day!). When we totaled the calories for the week, and the weight they would produce, she came out almost exactly her weight of 170 pounds. Each day she was teaching her body something different, one kind of abuse or the other. She was either beating herself up physically during the week, or beating herself up emotionally on the weekends.

This lead to her being overweight, having low self-esteem, and thinking that she could never succeed. None of this is true. As a commuter, she was constantly moving between these two different homes and not feeling 100 percent happy and comfortable in either one.

First, I had her eat 1,500 calories a day.

By adding in an additional 500 calories a day during the week, she had about twice the amount of energy. Why? Because, there was actually fuel in her tank. As a commuter, she was always running on empty. Not only was her week spent in an uncomfortable place, she had to push her body along because there was no fuel. Her 1500 calories includes at least 400-500 calories for breakfast. I cannot tell you how many faces I have seen light up when I start talking about the 500-calorie breakfast. Just like good vs. bad days, many people suffer from good vs. bad hours. (You may even be commuting back and forth each day.) They start their days off with the light toast and the watery nonfat yogurt, and then four hours later, their body is starving so they have two bags of chips.

I helped Cara cut out her excessive workouts, and just be active. Then, I told her, I did not care what she ate, but that it had to be real food. No, low-fat, nonfat or artificially sweetened foods packed with chemicals. (If your medical professional has recommended that you use these products, you should follow that advice. I am not your doctor, but I will make a strong intellectual argument for why, in my 30 years of experience, I have found that these fake foods do not work.) But back to Cara. In 24 weeks, she dropped 55 pounds and is now living full time in her dream house body.

Commuter Exercise:

If you are a commuter, here is your homework. Remember, we are just teaching our brains a new skill, the skill of maintaining our ideal self. Be consistent, driving home to your dream house every day can be a great feeling.

•Eat more during the week.
•Begin your new life on a Saturday; you are not a workplace.
•Work out less during the week, but be more active on the weekend. For example, a short Sunday morning hike.

Post the phrases:

•My body is not a job
•I am worth the effort

Add your own goals and motivational moments. You are teaching your commuting mind a new language.

Along the way, each of these people learned to eat and live for the person that they wanted to be, and they waited for their bodies to adjust. They had learned how much fuel their ideal house required every day. There is no need to learn anything else, ever! Along the way, you are learning to eat for your ideal person. When you get to your number you are done for life. You have successfully taught yourself to be this person, to live in your new ideal house that now becomes a home that you love forever.

Now that we have covered the three basic types, do you recognize yourself in one, or maybe all three?

Remember, we are discovering what we don't like about our current house so that we can choose our dream house and then make a permanent move. This is not a judgment about you; it is a fact-finding mission. The weight you are, how your body looks, and even how you feel about yourself, have nothing to do with who you really are.

Finding your ideal house

To find your ideal house and get the key you must teach yourself how. I'll show you how I did this and how I taught many others to do this too. Your body doesn't know the size you want to be, you must teach it. Let's get the address to your new house, the weight that you choose to be. Be specific. When choosing where you want to live, you may begin by choosing a town, but eventually you have to pick the individual house. I want an exact number. The more exact you are, the easier it is to get directions.

Here, is the formula:

- For women, multiply your desired weight by 13.
- For example, for me to maintain my 125 pounds, I eat 1,625 calories a day.

- For men, multiply your desired weight by 14.
- For example, my 200-pound 6-foot-4-inch husband gets 2,800 calories.

These numbers represent the calories we each need to sustain ourselves, in addition to an active lifestyle. By active, I mean that we walk each day, 10,000 steps, no crazy workouts in a Life in Synergy :-) It is important that the weight you choose be in the safe BMI range based on your height. Being underweight comes with as many risks and problems as overweight.

Check your ideal house's address in a BMI calculator online. Think of it as your fuel-burn rate. You may now understand why women gain weight once they get into a relationship. My husband's basic fuel mileage is almost twice that of my own. Often, because we view ourselves as equals emotionally, we think that this translates to physicality as well. It does not. I gained almost 10 pounds the first year we were married.

Why? Because I started to eat whenever he did. I was eating the calories to sustain his body, and his life, and not my own. I was acting like the thinker. Yes, I know it does not seem fair, and I know that you all have a friend for which this basic rule does not apply. (A friend that eats 5,000 calories a day and is still a size 2, who may be a classic decorator.)

This is the rule for the rest of us.

Choose who you want to be

Assess your current house's status, and define your ideal house, YOUR ideal house, not your friend's or a celebrity or your compromise weight, your IDEAL. It's not as complicated as you think. It's going to take some work, but I'm going to give you the tools, the road map, follow my directions and you will get there. Weight is a measurement. It's up to you whether you allow judgments around this measurement, or anything else, to govern you. The number has no power; it is just a number.

So here come the questions:

• *What if I exercise?* I don't care, still eat your number. We will get to exercise in-depth a little later.

• *What if I want pizza?* I don't care, eat your number in slices.

• *What if I get half way through the day and I only have 200 calories left?* I don't care, still eat your number.

Why is your number so important? You are teaching your body the size that you choose to be. By eating 1,625 calories a day, I am saying to my body, "Body, I would like you to learn to be an active 125-pound woman." I am teaching my body the language necessary to be this person.

"But Helena, that seems like a lot. I can only lose weight eating 1,200 calories." I have heard this too often. Your body really has not changed that much in the last 10,000 years. The only significant change is that some people have gotten slightly smaller palates, from no longer chewing meat off the bone, this is why so many of us had braces as kids. Your body has no idea that it is the 21st century, that there is a supermarket down the street and an endless supply of food.

It only knows what you teach it.

Now here is the magic: your body will learn. My body knows 1,625 calories is my fuel requirement. At 1,625, it is all done. It does not matter what food or alcohol is in front of me – at 1,625 for the day, I am done.

It is a learned behavior. But you have to be willing to learn. You have to take responsibility for your body, for the most important relationship in your life, the one you have with yourself. Sometimes, I have eaten close to my number at brunch, but then I'm done for the day. Let's talk about planning and pizza therapy.

On some Friday nights, my husband and I have pizza therapy. I eat an entire small pizza, sometimes right out of the box. Don't look at my pizza, do not ask me for a piece. It is mine! Oh, and don't forget the glass or two of wine. The total calories ends up being around 1,250. I remember my number – 1,625 – so for the rest of the day on Friday, I consume 350 calories. I wake up on Saturday still 125 pounds. No harm, no foul, no guilt. Am I at my optimal during the day on Friday? Probably not, but this is a Life in Synergy.

It is understanding how to fit in a full life, not just a managed one.

These are the plans that you need to make. My client Vanessa plans for a cheeseburger and fries on a Saturday. Steffanie makes room for cocktails. Once you understand how to fit all of these things in your life, you end up craving them less because you are not thinking and stressing about them all the time. Over time, pizza therapy happens less and less because my body, which has learned a whole new set of skills, is not craving that anymore. What happens when someone asks you to go out for cocktails after work and you do not have that many calories left?

This is where you get to make one of the most important decisions of your life. You get to ask yourself, "How important is it for me to love and respect myself?" Are interest and self-respect in yourself, or someone else, more important? Which direction is your pyramid pointed? Often we will choose the other people, just to wake up the next day with the same old thoughts about ourselves. This is an internal decision. You do not need to invite in the rest of the world, they will often try to sidetrack you.

Choose yourself! You are worth it 100 percent.

What happens if you made the choice to go out? You wake up and realize that you had three extra cocktails the night before, and you consumed far more than your number. On the road to a Life in Synergy, we all drive off into the gravel on occasion. Look around, take in the view and then get back on the road, right back to your number. If this keeps happening, maybe you picked a number that is too low.

This happened recently to my client, Angela, she picked 105 pounds as her goal. Though this would have still been in her BMI, (she is a bit over 5 feet tall) it was right on the borderline of being too low. We reassessed and made her goal 115 pounds, which was still within her range, but gave her an extra 100 calories a day and the freedom to enjoy her life as the sexy woman she is.

She can have a cocktail or a cookie and still feel amazing and love her body and her life. Be sure to not judge yourself along the way, but to take the time to learn from your actions. We are not here to judge, we are here to learn.

Your body is constantly learning your preferences, including your emotions. It has no idea that there is another option other than frustration. Your body thinks that frustration is essential for survival; it runs on that learned behavior.

Do not feed it. Teach your body about peace, empowerment and control. It will learn, and your whole life will change. Eat your number every day. I can eat my number in chocolate and still be 125 pounds.

I can eat it in fruit, I can eat it in protein, I can eat it in bread, I can eat it in ice cream. A calorie is a measure of energy. If something has 100 calories or 1,500 calories, that is how long that piece of food will give you energy to sustain your life.

Differentiate between calories and nutrition. One will keep you going, and the other will keep you going at full-speed. It is ultimately the combination of the two that will enable you to fully have your own Life in Synergy®.

Once you are fully fueled, you will have energy for your whole day. Imagine coming home from work and having the energy to play with your kids, or go out with your friends, or even to take an exercise class. This can only happen if you consume enough fuel to sustain the person that you choose to be.

But, Helena....

•But Helena, I don't want to count my calories.

You are responsible for the care maintenance and basic understanding of your body. You took the time to learn how to get dressed, brush your teeth and style your hair. You are responsible for learning how many calories are required to maintain you. Remember that your body is constantly learning. What does your body know now? Does it know that being overstuffed is your preference at every meal?

This is why people gain weight – they teach their body that full is not adequate and that they must be stuffed. The body learns this behavior and asks for the stuffed feeling every time you eat. Each year, you have to eat more and more to constantly feel stuffed. Learn a new behavior. Be in control. Love your body and your life.

•But Helena, counting calories is so hard.

This is the 21st century. There's an app for that.

•But Helena, I still feel hungry.

Yes, in the beginning you may feel hungry, probably more on the weekends when your body has learned that it has to overeat to survive (especially you commuters). Be in control of you. Love and teach your body. Your body knows that whatever you are teaching it is for survival, so you need to be responsible for teaching it your new preference. Being at peace with your body, being at peace with yourself is a Life in Synergy.

•But Helena, I can only lose weight on 800 calories a day.

If this is true, go to your doctor and have your thyroid checked. If that is not an issue, you are getting the calories somewhere. You need to be honest with yourself.

•But Helena, I want to lose 30 pounds this week.

You are responsible for teaching your body. When you teach your body starvation, it looks for the opportunity to feast. Your body is patient, it will wait, and suddenly all of your weight is back, maybe even more.

Learn the language of you. It has been my experience that people who learn to eat their number lose weight at about the same rate as a typical diet.

The difference is that because you are learning, it is much easier because you are at peace with what you are teaching your body. Think about when you where in school: if the class made sense, the learning was easy. Learning about you is the easiest and most exciting thing that you can do. The great added bonus, YOU ARE LEARNING AS YOU LOSE! When you reach your ideal house, you will have been learning to eat your number all along the way. The skill will be learned, for life! You will be done. Language learned, skill acquired, body produced, and life fully lived, your house of being will become a life long dream home.

•*But Helena....*

All of the buts are just your way of denying yourself success. You have learned to dislike yourself; it is what your brain and your body know. It is what your brain and your body believes is your preference. You do not have to live in your ditch with all your buts. Take my hand; I will pull you up. Learn the language of you, bask in the sunshine of your life and light up the world around you.

Write down your number in permanent ink. Send me your plan for your favorite foods and the words you'll think about to keep you on track. Live your life fully. Almost all of my days include a glass of wine.

What about yours? What rocks your world?

To-Do List For Your Plan

•Assess your house, and think about how you feel about it.

•Identify your ideal house. This is necessary before you can get the key.

•Remember your number and eat it every day.

•Make a plan that includes your treats.

•Refuse to abuse yourself :-)

•Know that I have complete confidence in you and your success.

Remember, until you really know and believe how amazing you are, I know and believe it for you.

Read on!

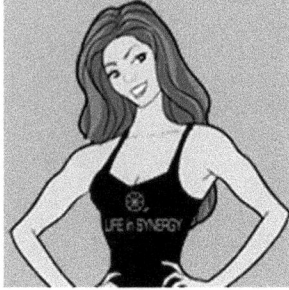

CHAPTER 3

TRIFECTA OF WEALTH

Animal fats, salt and sugar.

This is the first time in history that these three formerly hard-to-get commodities are not only readily available, but often less expensive than the formerly easy-to-find fruits, nuts, seeds and vegetables. It is as if you suddenly found yourself with an unlimited amount of cash, shoes and handbags, and then were told that using them are really bad for you.

It's not an easy thing to understand. They are all so amazing! And because of being historically in short supply, your brain and body have been engineered over time to seek them out and crave them.

The meat of the matter

Today, in many developing countries, access to animal protein can be restricted to less than once a month. All we have to do is hit the drive-through. It's a far cry from the days before animal farming, when every bite had to be hunted. I don't know about you, but I have a hard time even getting to the supermarket after a long day. Over time, our brains began to factor in this hardship and they learned to crave protein, to seek it out wherever they could.

Even up until a few decades ago, animal protein was expensive for the average family. Suddenly, in modern America, animal protein is available everywhere, for much lower prices. Your primitive body does not know how long this will last, so it craves it. Our bodies follow their instincts. What is your protein requirement? Protein should account for 20 and 30 percent of your daily calories. If you are like me, with a number of 1,625, this means 300 to 500 calories a day from protein.

That's essentially eating just one piece of chicken at only one meal. Sound tough? You're not alone. In general, we are all overeating our protein. Now, does this mean that I never have an 8-ounce burger or piece of steak? Of course not. They may cost me about 800 calories that day, but counting out burgers and steak completely would not be living a Life in Synergy. It just means that for the most part I limit my intake of protein to between 300 and 500 of my daily calories.

Where does protein come from? If it swims, walks or flies, it is a protein. But you can also get those nutrients from combining a legume, like a chickpea or a bean, with a starch. This is why many native cultures eat beans and rice as a staple—they're easier to obtain than a piece of steak. One of my clients, Jen, was eating a ton of protein every day, a tip she had read in a magazine. But every afternoon she was feeling sluggish and weighed down after lunch. As we looked at her habits and patterns, I noticed that almost every meal was filled with protein. We made only one change: removing chicken from her lunchtime salad.

Suddenly, she had a ton of additional energy that lasted all afternoon. Instead of weighing her down, she was raring to go. And the reduction of 350 calories a day lead to dropping almost 30 pounds in a year! Of course, let me say again, I am not your medical professional. If your doctor or registered nutritionist advises you to eat more than 20 to 30 percent of your daily caloric intake in protein, you should listen to them. They know you like I never will. I am just talking about basic guidelines set by the FDA and our history. I am teaching our brains how to eat, live and thrive in modern America.

But Helena, what about all of those high protein diets?

Well, some medical professionals might even tell you that those diets can be dangerous because they overtax your kidneys and put your body into ketosis, a way to metabolize fat instead of what our bodies are designed to metabolize, glycogen. This is not only unnatural for your body, it makes it harder to get much needed fuel to your brain and will often give you really bad breath. Then why do the high-protein diets work at first? Do the math! Your body can only handle so much at a time, so you experience a reduction in calories overall.

You can have the exact same reduction in calories if you are just aware, track your calories, and have a cookie, too! A Life in Synergy is a life that is filled with choice, happiness, success and options.

Stop managing and start living.

The Pillar of Life

Salt is a combination of sodium and chloride and, in its refined version, it is enhanced with iodine which was added to our table salt in the 1920s when it was discovered that a region of our country was deficient in this essential mineral, which caused thyroid disease.

Sodium is the most abundant electrolyte in our bodies. Contained within the plasma in our blood, it regulates the amount of water in our system and works in conjunction with potassium to create an electrical charge across the cell membrane that enables your muscles to contract. It helps to provide optimal nerve function, regulate your blood pressure, control the amount of water in your system and regulate your cells' absorption of nutrients. Whew, and we thought it just tasted awesome on chips.

Sodium is so important for our bodies and so essential to our lives as a means of preserving foods that it used to be a form of currency. The word "salary" comes from the word "sal" for salt. Not only were Roman soldiers often paid in salt, but many world economies, conquests of other nations and world-changing expeditions were funded by salt. (Columbus' sailto America might have been funded by salt.) Salt is a huge part of our world history.

Today, this gold standard is available everywhere and in everything. Most often it arrives in its cubic zirconium state, where it has been produced and refined through a series of chemical equations. This produces salt that looks more pure, white and uniform, but lacks all of the interesting flaws found in the originals. When you purchase naturally occurring salt, it will often be colored in some way due to the addition of other minerals in it. It is an ongoing joke in our house that I do not like salted butter, but I love natural cream butter on bread with a little natural salt on top.

The difference is amazing. First, the sweet butter is creamier in texture and the few sprinkles of natural salt enhance the flavor instead of overwhelming it. Ask any chef, salt is a huge flavor enhancer. It is also the best way to preserve something, to make it last longer. In the food business, shelf life is a major concern. How long can your product stay on the shelves in a store to be purchased by the consumer? Have you ever purchased a fresh loaf of bread or a baguette and then tried to eat it two days later only to find it hard as a rock? What about all of those decaying veggies in your fridge right now, or that leftover steak that turned in to a science project? These foods needed preservatives, a way to have staying power on your shelf.

This is a business. This is why so much of the American diet is filled with excess sodium. We go to the supermarket for our food, and purchase the packaged items that will last longer on our shelves. Many European cultures have different shopping habits that are directly linked to fewer weight and heart disease issues. They go to the butcher for meat, the farmers' market for veggies and fruits, and the baker for bread. All of these stores service a small community and carry a finite amount of product.

There is no need for extra preservatives because the food is going to be consumed fairly quickly. Have you ever watched one of those house shows for European properties? The refridgerators are so tiny! Now, it's obvious why we Americans love our supermarkets-convenience. Most of us are multi-tasking from the moment we wake up, to the last minute of our day. If your life is hectic, me tellling you to slow down and add trips to three different stores each day is not going to help. It will only make you more stressed. Living a Life in Synergy is about finding peace and balance, within our environment. Now worries, the supermarket is fine.

Just go into it armed with the knowledge that most of the foods that are packaged in a bag or a box have added sodium. You will look at the labels anyway to find the calories in your favorite foods, so take a moment and check out the sodium. How much do you need per day? The overall FDA recommendation is less than 2,400 mg per day. This is based on consuming 2,000 calories a day, so again, for me at 1,625, based on the FDA, I would need less than 1,900 mg.

This is gathering information about your life. Do it! Having the information leads you to informed decisions. If you have a favorite brand of frozen pizza that rocks your world, and the sodium content is through the roof, still grab a slice or two. On the days that you choose to get 80 percent of your calories from frozen pizza, spend the rest of them on fruits and veggies. Calories balanced, sodium balanced, life balanced. Armed with knowledge about how to best live in your environment, you have no option other than to thrive.

Let me eat cake!

Once a year, I decide that I am going to bake something from scratch. But Betty Crocker, I'm not. It takes me about four hours, and costs me about $100.

I never seem to have the correct ingredients or dishes on hand. My husband always says to me, "Why don't you just go to the store and buy a cake? It will cost you $10 and no time." But it is feeding more than just my craving for sugar, this is my primitive brain's moment of absolute wealth. I can use all of the sugar that I want, I must be royalty! Do you see an emerging pattern here? Baked goods used to be sweetened with honey long before sugar became readily available and in a processeded form like it is today. (Think about having to approach a hive of bees just to make a cake.) The development of sugar processing, as well as the change in taste buds, happened in the 18th and 19th centuries.

As this quick, storable source of simple carbohydrates became available peo- ple made fortunes and the slave trade began. All for sugar. Sugar is primarily derived from sugar cane, turned to syrup and then crystalized. It is a simple carbohydrate. This means it is a quick source of energy that your body converts immediately. No real digestion is necessary. This is why you crave sweet things when you are tired, even just mentally tired.

Your body knows that this will give you a quick boost to help you continue through your day.

Do you feel like you're constantly running on empty? Running from task to task, from problem to problem, from obligation to obligation. No wonder you crave this high-impact food all of the time. It is available everywhere and it's cheap. Seriously, how many stores have you been to this week with a candy display at the counter? For many Americans, money is one of the most stressful and emotional topics. Feeling stressed and tired mentally as you open your wallet? Hey, there is a candy bar to help you through this crisis.

This is basic marketing and business. It is filling a need that you have put out there.

Your ability to buy the candy bar that used to be reserved for only the most affluent is telling your subconscious brain that you are wealthy, that you are rich. Here is where being in charge of how you live your life and creating your own Life in Synergy comes in to play. You are now informed and aware. Are you eating the candy bar because you are really hungry or because you are stressed? Will eating the candy bar bring you peace right now and later today and tomorrow? Or are you just adding another bite of anxiety and stress in to your day?

Remember what we said about comfort foods. Happy feelings now could mean frustration later.

How comforting is that?

Look at how easy and affordable it is for you to get access to animal products and fats, salt and sugar. For many parts of the world, easy access to food is the journey to wealth. No wonder America is one of the richest countries. In our environment, wealth has become something different than it is for everybody else. What creates a Life in Synergy is the knowledge of how to live with our wealth without letting it destroy us.

We need to let our bodies know that stress does not need to be managed through food. We can understand how to live fully and not like spoiled, unhappy children that have been given so much but do not understand the value in what they have.

We can be grateful, and we can appreciate what our culture of food has to offer.

But we don't need to eat it all ourselves.

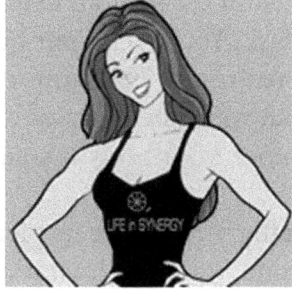

CHAPTER 4

THE TRIFECTA OF HEALTH

There's this miracle drug.

It helps with focus and concentration, a (ahem) regular restroom experience, better sleep, nicer hair, stronger nails, and leaping tall buildings.

Well, ok, not that last part, but it can reduce your chance of developing cancer and Type II diabetes.

And isn't that more exciting than mimicking a dude in red spandex? Sound too good to be true? Thankfully for all of us, it's not. It's simply the combination of water, fruits and vegetables working together to form the trifecta of health. Instead of following a diet that just tells you what not to eat, stick with me and the trifecta and you'll realize the secret of optimal health—the holy grail of a hot and healthy body.

Let's begin with part one, the essential element that can be found anywhere—water.

Grab a drink first

I often hear people say they are never thirsty. This is a learned behavior. When you are young, your body knows what thirst is, but then we start to manage it. You need to sit in class for an extended amount of time and then in a car, or at a desk. You teach your body how to do this and how to avoid needing the restroom. That, unfortunately, means you avoid liquids. We know that we all need water to survive, but how are you getting yours? Remember, your body is smart.

It throws a little tantrum after you ignore its pleas for a glass of water, so it throws a food craving your way, so at least it can get trace amounts of fluid packed into food. Here is the question: are you hungry, or are you actually thirsty? (And how much damage are you doing by "quenching your thirst" with a trip to the fridge?) Well, if you are craving that glass of water, you may actually be a bit dehydrated, which can happen even if you don't frequent deserts and road races.

Here are the signs:

1-Muscle Aches and Muscle Cramping

Whenever someone has a charley horse in class, I ask, "Did you get enough water today?" Most of the time, the answer is "no." If your back aches, or you wake up in the middle of the night with a charley horse, skip that pain killer and try an extra glass of water.

2-Feeling Tired

Do you crave that afternoon cookie or cup of coffee? I bet you're just thirsty, especially if you work in an office. (The air can be so dry.) But before you reach for the chips, stop at the water cooler. This happened to me just the other day. I mentioned to a client that I had been craving a lot of coffee, and he asked if I was drinking enough water. We all know he was right (and that even the teacher can need a push in the right direction from time to time).

I had been sitting, writing, and not drinking water all day. It was making me exhausted. My body thought, well, what gives us energy? Coffee. It put in a request (a.k.a. a craving) for it. Once I recognized this pattern, I grabbed the glass of water instead and the craving was gone. (Look who's the smart one now!) Now here is the great part, by teaching this to him a year ago, he was able to teach it right back to me when I needed the reminder.

Spread what you learn around, and you will be granted with help when you need it the most. Find your team!

3-Inability To Sleep

Sigh, I hear this one a lot. People who have a hard time sleeping are always worried about drinking water because they think they will have to get up in the middle of the night to use the bathroom. But your body needs enough water to restart fresh in the morning. Water is your body's fuel. Don't be that clunker of a car stalled at the red light.

4-Digestive Problems

Not going? Have a glass of water, nature's ideal lubricant. Having a hard time digesting? Have a glass of water. When in doubt, have a glass of water.

5-Confusion and Irritability

The organ with the highest concentration of water in your entire body is your brain.

So when you are dehydrated, it suffers the most. If you find yourself having a hard time understanding something or find that you are un-usually irritated, grab a glass of water. The fuel for your body is also the fuel for your brain.

6-Hunger

I know I mentioned this before, but it really deserves a second mention. If you do not give your body water, it will ask for food.

Have you noticed that all of these symptoms that I have mentioned sound like the ads on TV at night for the latest solve-everything drug. I know that you have seen them, restless leg syndrome, depression, insomnia, muscle aches...every- thing that they are advertising a drug for is actually a sign of dehydration. Let's be clear, I am not telling you to stop taking a medication, especially one pre- scribed by your physician. I am just saying that it is possible that many of these common problems can be solved with an extra glass of water.

Once my clients start drinking the correct amount of water, they cannot believe how profound the change is. My friend Joan used to reach for a cup of coffee every afternoon, but she started keeping a bottle of water at her desk instead. It wasn't long before she turned to me one day and said, "I cannot believe how much energy I have! My whole body feels completely different." Plus, the best thing about water is it's just one turn of the tap away.

How much water do you need? The recommendation is a ½ ounce for each pound of body weight. I need about 60 ounces. Now, I am talking straight water here. Not coffee, tea, soda, wine or beer. I will get into all of that when I talk about the food group, chemicals.

As you look at the symptoms of dehydration one at time they may not seem like much, but when you put them all together this could feel like a major illness. A little more water each day could make you focus better, be more productive at work, have fewer arguments, feel more energetic, eat less, get more sleep, and have a better-feeling body overall. Sounds like a miracle drug to me. If this came in a pill, it would proba- bly sell better than Viagra. Here is the caveat! Do not overdo the water. It's a ½ ounce per pound of body weight. Period. Too much water can be dangerous—it can swell your brain, and flush the electrolytes right out of your body.

A Life in Synergy is a life in balance.

Nature's Candy

Imagine me, for a second, wearing a headset in an infomercial. Hey folks, Helena Collins here with a new wonder drug.

• Do you crave something sweet to eat at the end of a meal?

• Do you finish your lunch, and then an hour later head towards the vending machine because you are hungry again?

• Do you worry about the toxins building up in your body?

• Is maintaining your blood sugar levels to fight off diabetes a concern for you?

Then have I got a great new drug for you!

• No muss, no fuss, it: comes in its own wrapper.

• Is filled with endless vitamins and nutrients.

• Will help reduce your chance of developing many diseases, including some cancers.

• Will detox your insides.

• Will help your cells regenerate, and your skin look better.

• Will help maintain your blood sugar levels.

• Will help you feel full longer.

• Is found in a single serving size.

• You can get yours today! (Shipping and handling not included.)

Nope, it's not another wonder drug.

It's an apple. Or any fruit, complete with the same basic nutrients packaged in a different wrapper.

Each of us knows how a two-year-old eats an apple. They are so excited, holding it in both hands, looking forward to every bite. As we grow up, where does this craving go? One day, instead of satisfying your sweet craving with an apple, you grab a cookie. Maybe you do it two days in a row. Come on, cookies taste great, right? By the third day, before you even think about the cookie, your body sends out a craving for one. (Remember from the previous chapter how your body knows that sugar is a hot commodity.) Now, your body has learned to swap the need for fruit with a craving for the cookie.

Your body has taken over and you are eating and living subconsciously. Before you know, the super fruit food group has disappeared from your diet almost completely. Go back, right now and reread what a simple piece of fruit can do for you. Almost weekly there is a new super fruit or berry being touted on the talk shows. I have to be honest, I really don't listen to any of that. I just eat fruit. Personally, I am a big fan of grapes.

They may be small, but they're chock full of anti-oxidants, that can prevent cancer, heart and nerve disease, Alzheimer's disease, and some types of infections. Plus, a nice bunch comes in under 70 calories, but still packs a punch with potassium, riboflavin, thiamin and vitamins A, C and K. Grapes may be one of my favorite fruits, but pick your own and then research their health benefits. You are going to be amazed, I guarantee it.

Instead of trying a new cookie this week, try a new kind of fruit.

The natural multi-vitamin

You've heard dieters who, even though they may be eating less, say, "I cannot believe how much energy I have!"
The reason is that dieting usually equals an increase in vegetables. A vegetable is your super vitamin, your stomach filler, your cancer preventer, your super-healer. They are life-changing power foods with a caloric cost of almost nothing. A cup of mesclun greens comes in at a whopping seven calories, while still feeding your body essential nutrients and vitamins. Now that can fit in anyone's life. And that is just the lettuce! I could spend and entire book talking about the health benefits, the amazing tastes and the variety of vegetables.

Do not be afraid of them!

I have a power lunch every day that consists of either a salad or vegetable soup. Not only does this ensure that I am getting these lifesavers in to my body every day, but it forces me slow down. One of the best things about soup or salad is that they require the use of a fork or spoon. No rushing through! (I can inhale a sandwich in six bites and then I am usually still hungry afterwards. Then my brain starts asking, Where are the chips?) By making my lunch choice a salad or soup, I take the guesswork out of my workday, and I am forced to stop and rest, which resets my brain and energy level for the afternoon.

I am energized by the influx of healthy vitamins and nutrients, not to mention the bit of self-righteous love I experience knowing I make healthy choices. The nutrients from a salad are more easily absorbed in to your system when they are accompanied by a little fat, which is why oil and vinegar (or, if you are me, blue cheese dressing) is so great on them. In fact, that was my lunch just a few minutes ago—a salad of greens, beets, olives, raisins, spinach, broccoli, peppers, pumpkin seeds, cucumber, celery, a hard-boiled egg and a little blue cheese dressing. Heaven!

You may not yet be in the rhythm of drinking water and eating fruits and veggies each day. No worries, school is in session. Over the next three weeks, follow the plan outlined below. It will teach your body not only to eat the trifecta of health, but to love it and crave it (and not cookies).

Don't attempt to go from zero to 60 with this. You have to learn a new way of being. When you force yourself to change too quickly, your mind and body just start looking for the end. By taking the time to learn a new way to live, your mind and body will learn to accept this as the new preferred behavior and they will naturally start to have healthy cravings. Get your health on! If you are already naturally exceeding the starting amounts, just stay where you are and wait until the plan catches up to you.

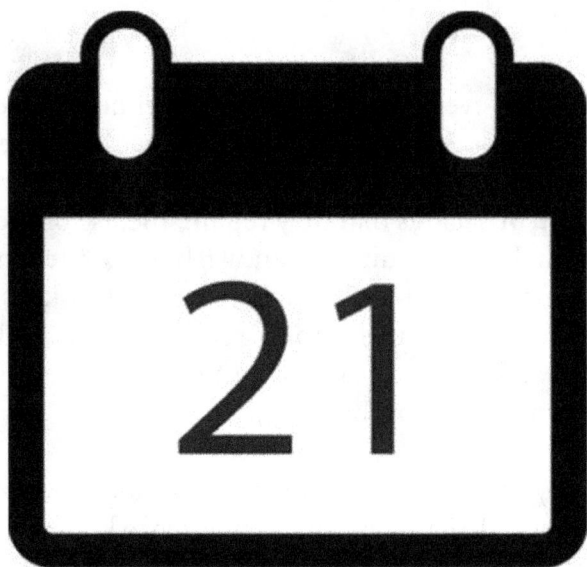

The 21 day plan to your future

Day 1: 16 ounces of water, 1 piece of fruit, 1 cup of veggies

Day 2: 16 ounces of water, 1 piece of fruit, 1 cup of veggies

Day 3: 16 ounces of water, 1 piece of fruit, 1 cup of veggies

Day 4: 24 ounces of water, 1 piece of fruit, 1 cup of veggies

Day 5: 24 ounces of water, 1 piece of fruit, 2 cups of veggies

Day 6: 24 ounces of water, 1 piece of fruit, 2 cups of veggies

Day 7: 30 ounces of water, 1 piece of fruit, 2 cups of veggies

Day 8: 30 ounces of water, 1 piece of fruit, 2 cups of veggies

Day 9: 30 ounces of water, 1 piece of fruit, 2 cups of veggies

Day 10: 36 ounces of water, 1 piece of fruit, 2 cups of veggies

Day 11: 36 ounces of water, 2 pieces of fruit, 2 cups of veggies

Day 12: 36 ounces of water, 2 pieces of fruit, 2 cups of veggies

Day 13: 42 ounces of water, 2 pieces of fruit, 2 cups of veggies

Day 14: 42 ounces of water, 2 pieces of fruit, 2 cups of veggies

Day 15: 48 ounces of water, 2 pieces of fruit, 2 cups of veggies

Day 16: 48 ounces of water, 2 pieces of fruit, 3 cups of veggies

Day 17: 48 ounces of water, 2 pieces of fruit, 3 cups of veggies

Day 18: 54 ounces of water, 2 pieces of fruit, 3 cups of veggies

Day 19: 54 ounces of water, 2 pieces of fruit, 3 cups of veggies

Day 20: 54 ounces of water, 2 pieces of fruit, 3 cups of veggies

Day 21: 60 ounces of water, 2 pieces of fruit, 3 cups of veggies

Want a FREE digital copy of the Nutritional Alignment Recipe Book: The Veggie Smile?

A great complement to Nutritional Alignment containing fun veggie facts and really great tasting recipes with their caloric info!

Just send a copy of your receipt to team@lifeinsynergy.com and we will send you your FREE Veggie Smile Recipe Book today!

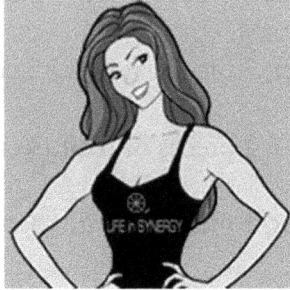

CHAPTER 5

CHEMICALS AND OTHER BASIC FOOD GROUPS

We all remember the food pyramid from grade school.

Filled with colorful images of fruits, vegetables, milk and grains, but where are the wine and cupcakes? Our food landscape has changed so much in the last 50 years with the mass production of food and farming as well as our ability to gain access to all kinds of products in easy convenient packaging.

I thought it was time to take a new look at the basic food groups.

Chemicals

No one ever addresses the chemicals in our diets, but come on, we are Americans—we love our chemicals. I personally break my chemicals down to two separate groups: natural and unnatural. Caffeine and alcohol are the natural chemicals we love to enjoy (glass after glass after glass), and the unnatural ones include artificial sweeteners, and pretty much anything on a label you can't pronounce, like dyes, preservatives and additives that act as stabilizers.

Remember, food manufacturing is a business. Food has to last longer, and look better, than is natural, so they need a little boost. (Consider additives the Botox of the food world.) The corporations work for a financial bottom line, and hope to make an emotional sale. By now, you've surely heard of the additive to ground beef that gives it color that is ammonia-based. But this isn't the only culprit. Let your imagination run wild and consider what might be in processed, prepackaged meat (there have been plenty of books and movies on this subject in the last few years). Now, does this mean I never eat a hot dog? Of course not; I love them. I just go in to it knowing that I am consuming a chemical, and account for it in my day. The same thing goes for my deli sandwich and the occasional plastic-wrapped cookie.

This is my body, and I have the free will to make an informed choice. But, as you begin to monitor your chemicals, you will be amazed how aware your body becomes. Processed foods can lose their appeal so quickly. Start small. If you use artificial sweeteners in your coffee to get rid of the bitterness, try adding a splash of cinnamon instead. It is natural, yummy, and it makes your coffee taste amazing.

As we get to taste bud alignment I will go into more detail about why artificial sweeteners pack on the pounds. Here's a teaser: Last year one of my clients lost 40 pounds. The only change I made to her diet was no Diet drinks. Eat for who you want to be. Artificial chemicals are for machines, not for humans.

My general rule is 4 to 6 natural chemicals a day. For me, that usually looks like two 12-ounce cups of coffee with cream for breakfast (3 chemicals based on an 8-ounce cup of coffee being one chemical serving), and one 5-ounce glass of wine with dinner. Make sure that you are aware of the calories in all of your beverages and account for them. Alcohol has 7 calories per gram. Now about the alcohol, let me share with you one successful client's vacation.

She went on the Margarita Diet while in Mexico. She planned ahead for her cocktails, supplemented them with fresh seafood and fruit, had a party filled vacation, and lost 2 pounds. By understanding herself, her true desire to party and her calories, she stayed on the road to her Life in Synergy. She came back refreshed, excited and really craving some healthy meals. The important part is that she did not return with the "get back on track" attitude. She stayed on the road and is now living her Life in Synergy. Plan for your chemicals. If you want a drink or two after work, don't eat any processed food during the day. Realize what they are and put a limit on them.

•*But Helena, I like to have 6 beers...*

Try drinking that much while staying within your daily caloric goal number. I promise it will be less than pleasant. What are you learning? You are learning how much alcohol the girl you wish to be can handle. You are that girl, you are just waiting for your body to catch up. You are teaching your body to live that life. (And couldn't you sacrifice a pint or three to get her on track?) Remember, the care of your body is your job. Never assume that somebody else has your best interest in mind. Businesses want to make a profit, but you need to know what products are best for you.

Here is a great example of a chemical vs. a real product experiment that I did on myself. I like cookies. I decided to compare the difference between a real bakery cookie and a processed chemical-filled cookie. The difference was amazing! The real cookie came in at 270 calories, and, of course, it was delicious. More importantly, after one I was satisfied, I could have forced a second one but it would have been an unpleasant feeling. Then I tried the packaged cookies with chemicals.

Two things happened, I was never satisfied, and I was never full. I could have eaten the entire box. (A little later we will discuss the difference between real food and manufactured and your brains ability to recognize it.) Unsatisfied and unfulfilled, I learned my lesson: The real cookie is better.

The beige building block

Carbohydrates come in three different categories—the sweet, the veggies, and the beige.

We know that the FDA recommends that 50 to 60 percent of your calories come from these food groups, so for me that would be about 800 calories. As we discussed earlier, a piece of fruit or a 1-cup serving of veggies comes in around 50 calories. That means for optimal nutrition 250 to 350 of that 800 calories will come from fruits and veggies, leaving 450 to 550 for the beige group. What is the beige group?

The starches, of course. The bread, the pasta, the corn, the potatoes, the rice. A staple of any nutrition program, and some of America's favorite foods. Starches are the foods that enabled us to grow as humans. Just look at the size of our ancestors, and you will see what I mean. We are much bigger than we used to be, mostly because of starches. They are relatively new to the human diet, easy to farm, rich in nutrients, and they come in at 4 calories per gram. But somewhere along the line, starches picked up a really bad rap.

How did starches become the bad guys? Science is mostly to blame. The science of processing broke our flour down to a fine powder, lacking fiber and substance. The science of preservation created trans fats, which made our food last much longer on the shelf and give soft white bread that smooth texture. The science of the deep fryer took the amazing potato and turned it into a fat-filled salt lick. (Enjoy those fries, just make sure they fit in your number!)

As a general rule, try to eat starches that look like a real grain. The darker the bread, the more filled with fiber and nutrients. Be aware of your calorie content for the day. Try to choose the starch in its original form. If you never eat whole grains, start with one slice, and put real butter on it! (So yummy.) You will be amazed how much more it will fill you up and how great it will taste. Think about your great grandmother's farm fresh bread straight out of the oven with real butter on it. Heaven!

•*But Helena, I can eat an entire loaf of bread...*

Remember that your number is your responsibility. Many of us learned to consume this food group way out of proportion. I have a theory and a way to learn a new behavior around this.

First, the theory. I do not think that our bodies recognize the yeast in bread as food. We have naturally occurring yeast in our system, so when we eat bread with yeast (especially when it is commercially produced) our bodies are not sure what it is, so they do not say when to stop. (Try eating unleavened bread. You'll find there is a big difference between eating an entire loaf of French bread and a bag of pita wraps.)

But if you have learned to be a starch-aholic, try the No Starch in March plan. I started this in my training studio about a decade ago. For the month of March, we ate no starches, no bread, potatoes, rice or corn. If it was beige, it didn't happen. Sure, it's extreme, but if you do this once, you'll cut down your dependence and never eat as many starches again. This is especially effective for the bread bingers out there. You are teaching your body to get it out of your system and that it's not a preference. Why March? Well, um, it rhymes. But that doesn't mean you're locked in.

Pick a month of your own and get started. (On a side note, if you do No Starch in March plan and you feel overly tired and sluggish, stop. You are not here to beat yourself up but to teach your brain and your body to function at the optimal levels.) Listen to your body and care for yourself.

The toppers

The Much-Loved and Maligned Fats!

Let's talk about fat, baby. Cream, butter, oil, love.

Here are the facts. For optimal health, approximately 20 to 30 percent of your daily calories should come from fat. My daily caloric intake of 1,625 (1,625 x 0.2 or 0.3) should consist of 325 or 488 calories of fat.

When it comes to calories, fats are a very dense form of them. (Eat a buttercream cupcake and you'll know what I mean.) Each gram of fat holds 9 calories in it, more than twice what a gram of protein or carbohydrate holds. A good rule of thumb is that there is going to be about

100 calories per tablespoon of fat. Because of their caloric density, fats make your foods last a little longer in your system, and help you feel satisfied longer.

Fats make your foods taste good. Think about bread without butter or salad without dressing. (Would life even be worth living? I'm kidding... Sort of.) They also contain health benefits, as many fats are anti-inflammatory. They naturally help you to decrease inflammation, the cause of many diseases, in your body. So how has fat gotten such a bad rap? Excess and science.

First the excess: Fats are toppers—butter on bread, dressing on salad, a little oil to sauté, a few seeds and nuts on a salad. (Note that nuts and seeds tend to be superfoods rich in anti-inflammatory properties, fiber and protein, but they're also quite high in fat.)

Somewhere along the line, we fell in love with fried foods and made fat our immersion choice instead of our topper choice. When this happens, you overload your fat quotient, get too many calories, and deaden your taste buds. Think of how butter coats a piece of bread, kind of like an oil slick on top, or bleu cheese dressing on a hot wing.

That is exactly what happens to your taste buds. It coats the flavor and takes it down a notch. Over time, your taste buds end up like one of those birds in an oil slick, coated and unable to fly or, in this case, taste. Then you eat more just to feel something. So, keep fats on top before they fill out your bottom.

Now, the science: You are going to hear me say this quite a bit, if your grandmother could not make whatever you are eating on her farm, it is not fit for human consumption. This includes not only products with trans-fats in them, but also all of the engineered low-fat and no-fat products.

They are not food.

Whenever they take fat out of a product, they replace it with chemicals, corn syrup or artificial sweeteners for taste. These culprits end up doing more harm than good. Recently after giving a lecture in which I recommended whole milk yogurts (170 to 200 calories) instead of the low-fat or non-fat alternatives (100 to 120 calories), a client called me because she could not believe how incredible the real yogurt was. Not only that, but it filled her up for a longer period of time. And after adding just a few blueberries to it, she didn't even want a flavored one. Because of this, her net caloric intake dropped.

The typical yogurt she had previously picked was not nearly as satisfying or yummy, so an hour later she was hungry again and looking for something else to eat. So instead of 170 calories from a whole milk yogurt, she would end up having 400 calories from the non-fat yogurt and then some toast with butter an hour later.

Food is not your enemy; it is your fuel!

Remember the rule with fats, if your grandmother or great grandmother could not make it on the farm, it is not fit for human consumption!

This means, Butter: Yes. Margarine: No.

Olive oil: Yes. Corn oil: No.

Nut oil: Yes. Vegetable oil: No.

Blue cheese dressing: Yes. Non-fat vinaigrette: No.

Whole milk yogurt: Yes. Non-fat yogurt: No.

By following this simple rule and by putting your fats on the top, you will enjoy every bite and end up eating fewer calories overall.

Eat for who you want to be, and use the yummy fats to keep yourself at your number. (I swear it's not too good to be true!)

Getting it all in

At this point, having taken a closer look at your wealth, your health, your chemicals, beiges and fats, you may feel a little overwhelmed.

It can seem like a non-stop river of information. Of course it is. You are an inter- esting and complex person, after all. But remember, you are more than capable of not only understanding all of this, but thriving!

You are in the process of learning about your Life in Synergy, of teach- ing your body your preferences, and understanding how your idealized life feels and works. All of these aspects are part of your unique life. Each day it is your choice to live the life that you want. This can make it all so much easier. You can choose to eat your number today. You can choose to get in your trifecta of health. You can choose which chemicals to indulge in. This is the best part of being an adult with choice.

Here is a great example, I received this email from a client of mine just a short while ago. By taking the time to learn about herself she is now free to live her life more fully. Amazing! (She talks about exercise. Don't worry, I'll get to that later.)

Hi Helena,

I just wanted to send a note because I'm not always able to chat with you when I come to the studio and I was planning to go to Kisses and Kudos [a party I had at the studio] on Wednesday, but something came up and I wasn't able to make it. So I thought I would send you my kudos via email at least.

I came to Life In Synergy when you first opened - I was working across the street at the time at an office in the Pru, doing a job I hated, but was too afraid to leave. Also at the time, I was punishing myself at the gym con- stantly. I'm someone that needs a lot of sleep (that just seems to be what my body wants) but I was forcing myself to get up at 5:30 a.m. every day to either run or go to the gym and do weight lifting classes because I got mad at myself and felt like I was "bad" if I didn't. I then would go on to work a long day at my job I hated, and then go home to a boyfriend who was selfish and completely took me for granted.

Running was certainly my punishment of choice - while I enjoyed it some- times (when doing it with a friend and chatting), for the most part my body hurt but I would yell at myself in my head, reminding myself of the cookies or big bowl of pasta I had eaten the night before and telling myself that I had to make up for it. At the time I fluctuated between 123 and 129 lbs, for the most part sticking somewhere around 127 or 128. I'm 5'5", so it's not like I was overweight, but I was still constantly unhappy with how I looked, and just felt generally....rounder, I guess, than I would have liked to be. I figured that it was just the way my body was meant to be and there was nothing I could really do about it.

I did Nutritional Alignment, honestly, for the goal of losing weight, and while I didn't really lose any (a few lbs. maybe), it did start to change the way I looked at eating, and helped me think more about how to add things in to my diet, instead of taking things out. And when I started to add healthy stuff in, there just sort of naturally wasn't room anymore for as much of the food that wasn't healthy for me.

Since starting to come to Life In Synergy, a lot has changed for me. I started using a pedometer (most days, too tough when wearing a dress!) I moved downtown and sold my car, so I walk everywhere now. I changed jobs and am back in school part time, moving in the direction of a job that will make me much happier.

I haven't run or lifted weights, or done a squat for about 2.5 years, and am happier with the way I look and feel now than I ever have been. I actually continued to lose a few more lbs., and while that wasn't my goal, it just sort of happened. I wasn't actively trying to lose weight, I was just more relaxed about everything, doing things I loved and thinking about eating to fuel my body rather than calm my nerves. My weight has been almost scarily steady at 114 lbs. for the 1.5 years. Like clockwork, every month at "that time" for a few days I retain some water and I go up to 116. But it's the same EVERY month, it's almost freaky. And while a few years ago I would have totally ripped myself to shreds for gaining 2 lbs. (crazy!) and not understanding why, I don't think anything of it now.

Anyway, that was a VERY long e-mail all to say that I can't thank you enough for helping me get to a point in my life where I feel relaxed about my body, I'm happy with how I look, and I no longer beat myself up over food or exercise. In fact, the other night I was really craving some choc-olate, and I sat down with a delicious piece of chocolate cake with cream cheese frosting and didn't think twice about it. I haven't felt deprived or punished in a long time now and it's fantastic! I enjoy life so much more. AND I sleep in when I want to!

Wow! I LOVE my job! By learning about yourself you too can have it all. Notice that during the first 30 days of the online Nutritional Alignment pro- gram, she says that she did not lose that much weight, a few pounds, probably 1 or 2 a week. Here is the kicker, while she thought she was not losing any weight what she was actually doing is teaching her body her number. Once realized her body continued to change until it reached it.

Put your plan in action and then sit back and one day you wake up changed, for life. No more thinking, stressing, worrying, anything. You can have it all.

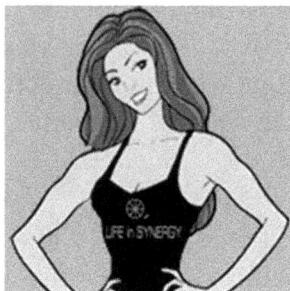

CHAPTER 6

GENDER - IT MATTERS

The very first year that I was married, I gained 10 pounds!

On my one-year anniversary, I was like, ummm... I am not really sure this is going to work. I love my husband completely but I would be totally dishonest if I said there was no resentment at his ability to eat so much and never gain any weight. My number is 1,625, and his is 2,800! Take a look back at the calculation of your number. Just by virtue of his increased muscle mass and the addition of testosterone in his body, a man of the EXACT same weight as you is able to eat more calories than you. My husband is 6'4" and 200 pounds. It is time to look at these facts straight on and embrace our differences, not bemoan them.

Realize that over time, our bodies have not evolved much from the early hunter/gatherer society. Societal roles influenced diets, as it does in the tribes that still exist in the world.

In these societies, the roles of each gender are stable, as are the types of food they eat, and the way calories are consumed.

The Women of the Tribe

Typically, the women of the tribe would be multitasking: raising the children, tending to domestic duties, and walking to gather fruits and vegetables that are the mainstay of the human diet.

How many women do you know who do not like to walk? We love it! It is in our nature.

Our muscle is predominantly slow twitch, made for long distances. Now, while on these long walks of gathering, we would be picking fruits and veggies and periodically snacking on them as we went along. (They're low-calorie fuel sources.) After our long walk, we would go back to the tribe where we would grind some wheat-like product into a flour, make some flat bread and have a little bit of the meat that the men would bring back.

This is ideal for women.

Lots of walking, with lots of fruits and vegetables, a little bit of bread and a little bit of protein. Not to mention the feeling of community, multi-tasking, snacking and looking around for pretty things. It used to be fruits, veggies, nuts and berries; now it's bags, shoes, home accessories and candles. (The former is better for our bodies AND our wallets.)

The Men of the Tribe

In these societies, men are responsible for hunting and heavy-lifting.

For a man there would be a lot of walking coupled with sitting around in the jungle (thus the love of the La-Z-Boy) followed by a quick burst of energy to run after and kill some sort of protein. At the site of the kill, they would consume the quick-to-perish organ meats and bring the rest back to the tribe. This is ideal for men.

Walking then resting, coupled with quick bursts of intense energy nourished with increased amounts of protein, fruits and vegetables and a little bit of bread. Remember the sharp difference in calories needed between men and women- extra muscle needs extra calories and protein to sustain. It also explains the love of the steakhouse. What have men replaced their spears with? The TV clicker of course!

As we look at the differences, it seems so logical, doesn't it?

Equal but different

My husband and I continue to marvel at our differences, even how we hear a conversation.
Just like the example of the tribe above, when I look for an answer to a problem, including what I would like to eat, I want to look at all of the options; I want to have a list of choices and change my mind as I go along. Often, all I am doing is voicing my mind's internal conversation. I am not looking for an answer, I am really looking to explore my mind and gather different thoughts just like I would as I walked along the path of a jungle gathering food.

The traditional hunters of the tribe want to get in, eat and get out. Simple and efficient. It is the combination of both of these styles that makes a complete and healthy tribe where everyone's needs are met. Just because you do something differently than someone else it does not make you better or worse, it just makes you an individual.

Putting yourself first

I really feel that it is important to point out that even though we are different in our needs calorically, it does not translate to the rest of our lives.
You may think that this is ridiculous to point out, but I have seen countless women sabotage themselves because deep in their hearts, they are not sure of this. As the most important person in your life it is essential that you understand how important you are. You have a unique role to play in this world. The rest of the people in your life are here to play a supporting role in your life as you are in theirs.

•But Helena, are you just asking me to be selfish?

No, I am asking you to be self-first. There is a huge difference. For me, it is the difference between being a spark and a flame. When you are self-first, you act as a spark—you are bright light that is able to light up the world around you. As you light each new spark by putting yourself first and shining, you end up with a huge bonfire of collective sparks. When you are selfish you act as a flame that just sucks all of the oxygen out of the room.

Let me give you an example:

A client came to me recently that was having a hard time finding time to take care of herself. The first thing I asked her was, "Who is the most important person in your life?" Oh, you should have heard the list. It was almost a novel: her coworkers who were not able to do their jobs, her mother who needed help, her sister who needed to lose weight, her kids who needed help with their homework and lives.

It went on and on and on. Her pyramid was flipped and that point was crushed into the ground. She had learned a pattern. Remember in the beginning when we talked about how you are not a lizard? You are constantly learning what to eat and adapting to your environment. Well, the same holds true in how you manage your life. This woman had learned that in order to survive, she had to help everyone around her and often "help" meant take over for them. Now, on the surface this may seem like she was really just helpful all the time. But by constantly being there for everyone else, she was not there for the most important person in her life: herself.

She was also preventing those in her life from learning about themselves. I gave her homework for the month, like I have done with many others like her. For an entire month, unless the question or the need of the other person was really her responsibility, I asked her to respond, "I don't know." Instead of jumping in and just taking over, she allowed the people in her life to work for themselves. A wise person once told me, "You know, people will do things differently than you and that is okay." What an amazing lesson to learn. As this woman allowed the people in her life to work for themselves, all of this free time appeared and with it

71

she was able to take care of herself.

Here is the spark: as she was able to take care of herself, those around her were inspired to take care of themselves. She became an inspiration for them as opposed to taking responsibility for them. This made all of the interactions with all of the people in her life more meaningful. Her coworkers noticed a change in her attitude because she was not feeling burdened by them and when they legitimately needed her help she was happy to give it and they were more grateful for it. Her mother began spontaneously doing more for herself and felt better about her life.

Her sister was inspired by her weight loss and starting doing the program herself and her children started doing more for themselves, asking for more fruits and vegetables without badgering and her time with her children had become more joyful. All because she put herself first.

I cannot tell you how many times I have heard from moms who started Nutritional Alignment for themselves and then all of a sudden their husbands are asking about their numbers and their kids are asking for more fruits and vegetables. When you are the spark of your world you light up the world around you and there are no burdens to bear and no fights to be won (with others or with yourself).

Think about how much free time you will have every day just by not worrying about what other people are thinking of you. Think of all you will accomplish. In my world, as each of you learns to love yourselves, learns how important you are, you increase the peace and happiness in your world and in mine. I am not interested in competing; I am interested in each individual finding their own happiness, their own peace, and then utilizing that peace and happiness to spark those around them.

The couples plan

Plan, plan, plan.

You are the most important person in your life. Have a plan to get it all in.

Pizza therapy on your list?

Know how many calories you have going in to the evening, and know exactly what you're ordering as you eat, drink, and commence with the merriment. I have found an easy plan for dinner is to have an appetizer, and either give half of my entree to my husband who gets an extra 1,200 calories a day, or have the waiter pack it up before it comes to the table. Then, instead of taking home half-eaten food, you have a fresh extra portion to go. Your body, your food.

You are not here to eat what your kids do not want. You are the most important person in your world. Treat yourself that way. It's important to remember that you're learning. In the beginning, I had to spend the time to learn the skills, but now I own these skills and my body has learned when to stop, when I have had enough, when I have reached my personal fuel mileage for the person that I LOVE to be, now that my house of being is my ideal home!

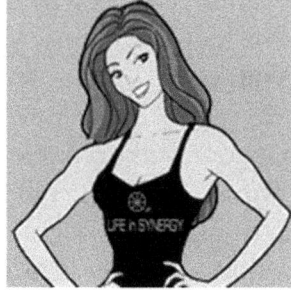

CHAPTER 7

LEARN TO CHOOSE FOOD THAT YOUR BRAIN RECOGNIZES

Doesn't my brain recognize everything that I am eating? (Yes, I see that pink cupcake with the adorable frosting design…that's the problem.)

Well, you would be surprised.

Your brain is constantly learning, especially when it comes to making the best choice for you when a buffet line has everything from cinnamon buns (extra icing, please!) to an omelet with egg whites.

Using your brain's existing hardwiring, plus a few extra healthy tips, you can make food choices and feel satisfied after every meal.

Your primitive self

We operate our lives from two separate states of consciousness. Your primitive self can also be called your subconscious brain. It's the part of you that takes control and moves you through life without you having to think much of anything. We experience this part of ourselves in a conscious way at times. Have you ever driven somewhere but not remembered the trip there? This is because your subconscious brain and your body understand the mechanism to drive and they just take over, almost as if you're asleep. Your conscious mind eventually realizes, "Hey, driving is my job!" and for an instant, you are aware of your two separate states of mind.

It's like learning to walk. As a toddler walking requires participation from our conscious mind. Our mind has to teach our brain how to fire the nerves that place one foot in front of the other. Once we learn it though, off this task goes to the subconscious mind, to be carried out without conscious thought for the rest of our lives (except, perhaps, when we wear a new pair of heels).

Just like keeping our heart beating and our lungs breathing, this subconscious mind can also take over when it comes to eating. This includes what we eat, how much food we think we need and how full we think we need to be after every meal. These are all behaviors that our subconscious mind has learned, but there is always time to teach that old dog some new tricks. If you teach your subconscious that every time you eat, you need to feel stuffed, it will not be satisfied until your pants are about to bust open.

But because that waistline is sure to expand (thanks, in great part, to the wonder of spandex), you will have to increase the amount of food you eat over time to still get that same feeling of satisfaction. Then one day, 10 years later, you wake up and you have gained 50 pounds. Why? Because you are running the eating-means-I-have-to-feel-stuffed program. It is time to learn a new program.

What your subconscious brain knows right now about food

Let's look at what our super computer came installed with already as far as food recognition and portion control. You wake up in the morning and you are hun- gry, how many hard-boiled eggs do you want? On average most people answer one or two.

You wake up in the morning and you are hungry, how many eggs do you put in to an omelet? On average most people answer three or four and that does not even include all of the things that they will add in to their omelet, like cheese or veggies. In addition, when you think of hard boiled eggs you pretty much think about the egg itself, no home fries, no toast, etc. But the omelet, that comes with a whole host of extras.

Why are these two so different?

When you look at a hard-boiled egg, your primitive brain knows what it is. It knows how you will feel after eating it, and it knows how many it needs, so it self-regulates. Once you process the egg by scrambling it (yes, I said process), your brain is not quite clear what it is seeing. It will then run the omelet program, which it knows comes with home fries and toast, and that is exactly what you will crave.

Think about the difference between a piece of steak and a burger. The process of grinding the meat sends your brain in to a new program. You have left the original base programming that knows that a few ounces of steak is plenty and moved on to a program called burger that comes with cheese, a bun and fries. Processing is any change to a basic food from its original state. We all know that one apple is a single serving, but how much juice or applesauce should we eat? Think about the differ- ence between whole milk and skim milk, an orange and orange juice, a piece of grain-filled bread and white bread. The farther away from the original, the more you have to engage your mind to create a limit. This is why you can eat an entire box of processed, preservative-filled cookies and still be hungry. Your primitive, subconscious brain that sets natural limits has no idea what that food is, or that it even is food since unnat- ural chemicals are not even on the human consumption list. It does not engage, requiring your conscious mind to set a limit. (And that one cannot always be trusted. You remember your hair in the 80s, don't you? Case in point.) I am not saying that a burger is not great.

I am just saying that the more you process your food, the more conscious you have to be, and the more you have to learn about your own limits for each food. How many pre-shelled or chopped walnuts, complete with added fat and salt, would you eat (or absent-mindedly shovel into your mouth while watching TV) compared with walnuts still encased in their shells?

The shells are a built-in limit, making you really work for the food, therefore stay conscious about what you're actually eating. If you do not want to spend the time to think and learn about every bite you take, keep it real, whole and as natural as possible.

Pretty soon, your conscious and subconscious mind will work together to help you on your way to living a Life in Synergy.

Using your conscious mind to learn

It is only through our conscious mind that we are able to learn and create the life that we want to live.

Your conscious mind is where your personal responsibility is found, the part of you where your judgments are made, and your learning is accomplished. Learning to know how to eat for your environment and the person that you choose to be is no different than learning how to walk or read.

Just because you are an adult does not mean that you do not have things to learn. Learning, especially about yourself, is not only rewarding, it is fun. And it is also your responsibility.

Expanding your awareness

The first thing we all need to do when beginning a new class is realize it is just that—new.

When it comes to food and eating, we place all kinds of judgments on ourselves before we even begin. "I have no willpower," "my genetics are different," "my life is too busy right now," "it is too hard." Realize how all of these statements would sound if your were walking into a math class.

You would instantly recognize that you are psyching yourself out before you even begin. Just because this is your body does not mean that you should already know everything or else you are flawed.

It just means that you have not taken the time to learn how to live in your en- vironment, or to engage your conscious brain to teach your subconscious brain how you choose to live. As you look back at what we have covered so far, you can see how each of the lessons have lead to this moment.

You need to learn to crave fruits and vegetables, you need to learn to crave the correct amount of water, you need to learn what your personal gas mileage is and how you fit things like alcohol, pizza and nachos in to your life. As you apply yourself to learning about you, your life begins to take shape.

Instead of following a diet (another short-term management program) you learn what your life looks like, and as you do, your body will teach you right back. Here is a great example:

A client of mine has been doing Nutritional Alignment for approxi- mately a year, on and off. She would eat her number for a while and then blow it off. Despite this on-and-off approach, she has lost 15 pounds and all of her blood work that was pre-diabetic and border- line high cholesterol had moved in to the normal range. Her doctor is thrilled, but she is still not living her ultimate life. With a new dedica- tion to herself, she really started monitoring her number and trifecta of health every day. Suddenly she found herself, out of the blue, craving spirulina, or dietary supplement drinks and even seaweed salad! This was definitely not something that she would have ever thought of eating or drinking before.

As it turns out, she has a thyroid issue, and spirulina and sea vegetables are great for that. Filled with iodine, iron, vitamin A and other trace minerals, they are like thyroid super foods. Here is the important part. By spending time thinking about herself, consciously eating her number and following her trifecta of health, her body started to self-regulate.

Her mind and body became active in her ultimate health. Because we only know a fraction of what our brains are capable of, our job is to activate and apply them to creating our ultimate life, understanding that our life is our conscious choice. Hoping that someone else will do it for you will never work. Realize that this is just a class for participation and learning, and take the emotions out of it except, of course, for pride.

Review:

•Eat your number
•Learn about your trifecta of health and consume them every day
•Learn about your choices so that you can make informed ones
•Stop judging and start learning!

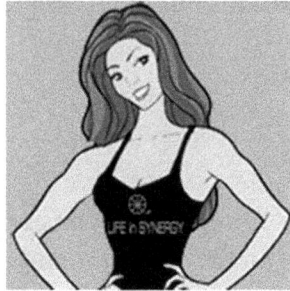

CHAPTER 8

UNDERSTANDING THE ROLE OF EXERCISE

I have been in the fitness industry for more than 30 years. I have won awards, been featured in all kinds of publications and have been seen on television numerous times. I have developed my own Synergistics Fitness Method® that gets people in shape in half the time of other workouts, and teaches them how to change their body shapes through conscious communication.

I make my living from exercise. Having said all of that, I know that the science of exercise lacks basic critical thinking, and that the fitness industry is partly responsible for the obesity crisis in America. (Unfortunately, that's no joke.)

First let's start with all of the rules:

You need cardiovascular work almost every day; you need strength training work three times a week; if you are a woman, you can never put muscle on your body; when you reach a plateau in your weight loss, you need to increase your workout; when you are able to lift a certain amount of weight, you should increase it; you need to run to burn stomach fat, even though you hate it and it kills your knees.

If only you could learn to move like a ballerina or stand on your head like a yogi—then you would be fit.

Are you kidding me? When in all of this do you get to live?

Life is not about worrying about when you will fit in your 2-hour workout, or constantly stressing about your next meal. It is about expressing your unique qualities. All of these rules are just business and hype, continuing in the survival-of-the-fittest mode.

It is time for us to evolve.

What is exercise

Exercise comes in two parts: activity and thoughtful movement, which brings your body back into alignment, optimal function and joy. Activity is the amount of movement each day that you should get as an active human being. But first you need to realize that there is a difference between an athletic endeavor and a human endeavor. Like I said, I am in the fitness industry and have been for more than 30 years. I am a scientist and a teacher.

Believe it or not, I am not an athlete. Yes, my body looks great and feels great, but I do not want to and do not need to spend hours every day just to look like this. That is a misinformed myth. Yes, I said it. You do not need to go to the gym every day to look and feel great. (And this is coming from someone who owns her own studio.) In fact, going to the gym every day may prevent you from losing weight, make you dislike the shape of your body, and make you more prone to injury. (This is often the dirty secret in fitness. Many fitness professionals are in chronic pain, and do not love their bodies.)

For me, time spent in the gym is to increase my brain's communication to parts of my body, not to beat myself up. A Life in Synergy is not about just a few looking great, but all of us looking great and loving our lives, not forcing ourselves in to submission or accepting that others are better than us. Each of you is amazing; my goal has always been to help you realize it.

Fight or flight, also known as the Cardio Myth

When you increase your cardiovascular output, you increase your caloric output.

If you want to lose weight, you just have to do some sort of cardiovascular workout every day. Seems simple enough, right? But cardio isn't the only thing that gets your heart pumping. Even with feelings like stress or first-date nerves, your body starts to produce hormones like cortisol that help you to retain fat and increase the production of adrenalin and endorphins. Then, your appetite increases. This is part of your fight or flight reaction. Picture yourself living in a primitive village. As an adult woman, why would you need to run every day? Is the lion attacking the village?

Is there a raid that you need to escape? And, if you are living in a stressful situation like this, you better force down as many calories when you can because you may have to run away from the lion again tomorrow. Sounds dreadful! There is no difference between this scenario and forcing yourself to run or get on the elliptical machine every day (especially since I'm pretty sure you're all set on the wild animal front). The best piece of fitness equipment you can buy is a $10 pedometer—not so that you can go on a 5-mile walk and then sit around the rest of the day, but so you can learn to be active. This is what is missing in modern day society. We have taught ourselves to sit, to take an escalator, to send an e-mail instead of getting up and talking to the person in the office down the hall, to drive around for an extra 10 minutes burning gas to find the closest parking spot instead of just walking to the store. Our bodies are designed to be active. When you are active, and when you are walking, your body produces natural anti-inflammatory agents that fight disease, your brain receives extra oxygen that improves problem solving, and your bones maintain their density better as you achieve the correct amount of impact with each step. You do not need special shoes, a specific outfit or a plan for your time. This is real fitness.

In Boston, you can spot the Life in Synergy girls anywhere. They all have pedometers on. Each and every day, in addition to eating my number, I walk 10,000 steps. Every day. Sometimes those steps happen on a pleasant walk in the woods with my husband; sometimes they happen during commercials in front of the TV; sometimes they happen as I walk from the train to my office, out to lunch, around work and back to the train.

The important thing is that I am just naturally moving throughout my day. I am not power walking or stressing about it. I am just moving. Now, if you are not moving at all right now, start with 2,000 steps a day and gradually increase each week until you get to 10,000. You are not going to believe how great you are going to feel. In my Walking and Water program we do this over 8 weeks. You get a water bottle and a pedometer, the two most important pieces of health equipment, and I teach you the 6 minutes of stretches that I do every day to keep my body healthy and aligned. And that brings me to the other part of exercise: Alignment.

What you don't like about your body is not a fitness issue, it is a communication issue

Another one of the myths of exercise: You cannot spot reduce, or target just one area for improvement.
Well, then I must be hallucinating because I help women do it every day. This is when time spent on yourself really pays off. When you do not like a part of your body, I guarantee it is a communication issue, and not an exercise one. For my whole life, I hated my butt and thighs. People actually used to call me Thunder Thighs. In an effort to change them, I did every cardio workout, I squatted, I lunged, I did Pilates, I tried yoga. You name it, I tried it. The problem with all of this is that I was just going through the motions and not thinking. Even if the exercise looked great, I was not thinking about which muscles should be working I was thinking about the exercise.

We learned in the last chapter the difference between our conscious and subconscious brain. Never are these two parts of our mind more in play than when we move. When you go to the gym and do an exercise, your brain has no idea why you are doing it. It just looks at the task at hand

and then sends signals to your body through your nerves to complete the task. End of story. Remember, you are not a lizard, so throughout your life, your brain has learned to communicate with your body to complete the jobs that it needs to do in order to survive. Combine this with your genetics, the subconscious programming that you came in with, and you end up the shape you are today.

In order to change the shape of your body, you need to work on your communication, not the exercise. In order to change the shape of my butt and thighs, I needed to learn how to communicate with them more effectively, which involved learning their language. I learned about the action of the muscles involved, where the muscles are attached, and which bones and joints they affect. Once I understood this, I could learn how to use my conscious brain to talk to my body. What does this mean? First, I thought about what I was specifically unhappy with and then I thought about why I was unhappy. Let me give you just one example of what I have discovered.

No matter how much I ran, squatted and lunged I still hated my butt. It was always a little flabby and covered in cellulite, even when I was 110 pounds and working out hours every day. Where was my communication off? As I looked in the mirror I realized that my hips were almost in a constant state of flexion. Do you have that sweep in the front of your thighs like I did? Now, I knew that my hip flexors (iliopsoas is the muscle) flexed my hip and my butt (gluteus maximus) extended my hip, I knew that these two muscles worked in opposition, so I thought about what I was thinking every time I ran, squatted, or lunged. I was thinking about putting my foot forward or bending, in other words, I was asking my hip flexors to flex all of the time, not to mention every time I sat down in a chair. I did not even know how to communicate to my butt.

I was working out through my subconscious mind only. It was time to go back to basics. I laid down on the floor and tried to just squeeze my butt, seems simple but boy was I trying to get others to help, I would push down with my feet, squeeze my hands, tense my shoulders. My brain was unclear how to just talk to my butt. Even if I bent my knees I noticed suddenly that I was pushing down with my feet or using the muscles in my back to lift up. My butt was talking one language and my brain another. Knowing that I am the most interesting, amazing person in my world, I persevered. Instead of doing exercise, I developed a system that teaches my brain how to improve communication with body parts that are lacking and exercises to teach the over worked ones how to relax.

Remember, the part of your body that I am most interested in is your brain. I just had to take the time to learn about the most important person in my life: myself. Not only do I love the way my butt looks now, but instead of being a source of frustration and anger for me, it is now a source of comfort and inspiration. When I am having a tough day all I need to do is teach Lean Legs and I am instantly happy. Not only that, but when I hated my thighs and butt, they hated me right back. I was living with chronic back and knee pain, (those tight hip flexors originate on the spine and where constantly pulling on my back) now, I'm pain free.

A Life in Synergy is a life of happiness and peace.

Many people will say that women's triceps are doomed. Once we start to age, it's all over, and we'll be forever confined to a life of flab. This is another example of miscommunication. Look at any woman walking down the street and you'll realize that throughout our lives, we are almost constantly contracting our biceps every time we carry something like a purse, or a bag of groceries, or a child. And now combine that with the amount of time we all spend typing. As I look down at my arm, even though it does not seem like I am doing anything, my brain is sending a signal to my biceps to contract against the force of gravity. Over time, your biceps become stronger and stronger, and the opposing triceps muscle group gets flabbier and flabbier. By the time you are 60, flabby arms make their appearance, but this does not mean that you cannot change.

I have a client that started at Life in Synergy at 65. Five years later she has the most amazing body, she is in the best shape of her life, and she loves how she looks. Instead of wasting time in the gym exercising your strongest muscles, spend time working on muscles that are overlooked and underused. Wherever you are flabby, you are lacking communication. So start with those spots the next time you're in the gym. There is a picture of me flexing my biceps on my website, and I have not done a single biceps curl in more than 20 years.

Loving your body

Here are just a few of my favorite quotes from clients:

"Since I stopped running I have dropped two dress sizes."

"I know I did not believe you before, but since I injured myself and could not run I have not been hungry and I have lost 10 pounds."

"I cannot believe how learning about my stomach has changed my shape, I spent an hour in the car just contracting it and feeling it, and my next workout was amazing and it looks better in just one week."

"I have so much more free time now, I started taking a class in the evening and I have never looked better."

"Okay, not only do my legs look better but my knees do not hurt for the first time in years."

"My husband said there was no way I could get in better shape working out one day a week until he walked in when I was getting dressed and said, 'Oh my God, your abs look amazing.'"

"I cannot believe how much better I look and feel now that I stopped running, started walking and just do a few workouts a week."

"My husband and I go for a walk together now every night. It is such a great way to spend time together and since I am not getting on the elliptical machine, I am less hungry and my husband said my butt is looking great. Thank you!"

I am not interested in competing, winning or survival of the fittest.

As each of you learn to love your bodies and your life, you are increasing the love in my world and your own.

Having your plan

I know exercising, like eating, can be emotional. But it's really just science.
Start by taking a deep breath. I mean it, right now, as you read this. Breathe in, hold your breath for a moment, and exhale. Repeat three times.

Okay, now that you are relaxed, get yourself a pedometer and go. Start without a plan so that you can get a better understanding of how your activity level is already.

For example, when I first started wearing a pedometer, I realized that my activity plummeted on Sunday, when I barely walked 2,000 steps all day. (What can I say? We all know Sundays and couches go hand-in-hand.) Now that I have learned that about myself, I start my day with a brief 20-minute walk. This sets me on an active path for the rest of the day. I learned about me and then made a plan for my life. If you are not moving at all, make your goal 2,000 steps a day and then increase your steps by 200 a day until you reach the goal of 10,000 steps.

Get your kids involved, they LOVE pedometers. If it is a family goal, it will be that much easier to accomplish. When you need a break, make it a walking break. Stressed about a problem at work? Take a walk. Someone was telling me the other day about the CEO of a major healthcare company that holds his meetings while walking. Not only does the action of walking increase the oxygen to your brain, helping your problem solving skills, the idea of two people moving in the same direction puts the subconscious brain in the mutual agreement mode, so they are both walking in the same direction for the solution. Having a hard time communicating with someone? Go for a walk together and try this powerful CEO's solution. If you love to watch TV, make the commercial breaks a walking break.

I know it is exactly 200 steps from my living room, through my kitchen, around the dining room down to the family room and back. Sometimes I do the commercials just marching in place. Every step is a step against the force of gravity. They all count, they all increase the amount of anti-inflammatories in your body, and each and every last one contributes to your health. Don't stress about finding that perfect parking spot. Just pull in and park at the end of the lot, get your shopping in, spend less time parking, and get your steps in. Do you know someone who works when you are home who has a dog? Offer to take the pooch for a walk.

Need to talk to a coworker? Get up and walk to their office instead of sending an e-mail, not only will you get your steps in, but speaking face-to-face will improve your communication skills. Need extra steps at work? Walk the extra block to the next sandwich joint or coffee shop. Take up line dancing, start a walking club or a professional window-shopping group. The possibilities are endless and completely customizable to your existing lifestyle. Post your favorites on the Life in Synergy Facebook page and inspire the world with your fitness.

As far as learning about how to communicate with your body to change your shape...if you are not in Boston and cannot make it to my studio, no worries, help is on the way! I am producing 5-10 minute online videos for each part of your body. Pick just one area to improve, who knows where the journey to learn more about yourself will lead. Every one of the teachers that works for me started as a client. Learning about themselves was so interesting that they decided to learn even more science and now they pass it on to others. Not exercise, science. There is a reason that my intensive training classes are often filled with nurses, physicians and physical therapists but also populated by artists, lawyers and moms.

I am teaching science in everything that I do. Being the geek that I am, I know that science can be fun and exciting especially the science of you.

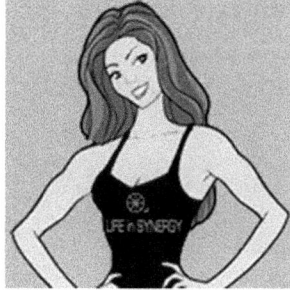

CHAPTER 9

EATING FOR PEACE

What do we really want? It's deeper than just leaner legs or flatter abs.

It's a feeling you look for when you try to put on your favorite jeans or bikini come summer time. The answer is peace. We all want to be at peace with ourselves, our lives, our bodies, our relationships and our communities. Think back to what I said earlier, about how your entire day can be ruined because a particular outfit does not fit or the number on the scale is not what you expected or wanted to see. We can end up lashing out at others because we are not happy with ourselves.

Peace begins with each of us.

Remember the pyramid from the beginning of the book, where you learn to put yourself on top.

Where are you looking for answers?

Here is a gentle reminder, you are the most important person in your life.
Now how do we fuel the self-esteem of this great person in your life?

Too often, we look for it outside of ourselves:

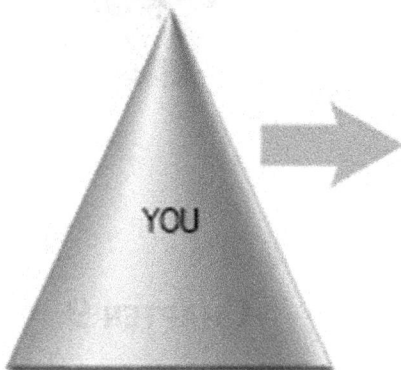

What do you think about this shirt, these jeans, this guy, my job? Have you asked these questions of others? Of course you have; we all have. We ask these kinds of questions because we are not clear in our own minds. We do not have a clear vision and the opinions of others can help to clarify our own thoughts and choices.

Their experience can help to guide us to the right choice for us. Here is the kicker though, have you subjugated your opinion of yourself to what others think or even what you think they may think of you? This kind of outward thinking can stop us cold in our tracks, preventing us from really expressing who we are and what we are able to contribute to ourselves and to the world. Part of learning to put yourself in the right place in your life is learning to fuel yourself, to understand yourself and to allow the radiance that you have built shine out to light up the rest of the world.

This is how peace begins with each of us. How does all of this relate to eating? Comfort foods and peer pressure. Just like with exercise, your conscious brain is teaching your subconscious brain different preferences, and this is never stronger than in these two categories. Many of us have taught our subconscious brain to feel bad about ourselves. So often in fact, that feeling bad about ourselves has become the norm. How many hours have you spent on the phone with your friends complaining or listening to them complain about themselves? The negative has become our default pattern of being.

Think back again to the beginning of the book, the three personalities, the thinker, the decorator and the commuter. It does not matter which type you are. What matters is that they all have the same thing in common. All are finding ways to stay unhappy and unsatisfied. This is the addiction we all share—the addiction to disliking ourselves.

The other day I was in the studio and was talking to a client, "Hey Stacey, I see that you are back to eating your number." I could tell that over the past six months, she had stopped eating her number and had gained 15 pounds. But now she was back on track. She explained she had been going through a tough time, and had fallen off the health wagon. "Yeah, good for you!" I joked. "You found a way to have a hard time in your life, and wake up each day disliking yourself at the same time." In that moment her eyes lit up, "You are so right, I never thought about it that way!" We all do this, but we're not aware of it at the time. We fall back in to the ditch of our problems and then run the "My Life Sucks" program, which comes complete with comfort food, weight gain and decreased self-esteem. Imagine going through that same tough time and each day getting on the scale and loving your body and yourself. It makes everything that much easier to deal with.

When I pointed this out to Stacey, it was not to make her feel bad, but illuminate a pattern so that she could learn more about herself. Each time we go through something like this and learn from it, we are getting to know ourselves better. This can be the most profound learning experience of your life—you learning about you. There is no room for judgment here in a Life in Synergy, just learning.

Let's meet another client. Meg is a smart, pretty, fun-loving girl, she just doesn't really know it. She spends a lot of her time thinking about what others are think- ing about her.

Often, at the end of her work day, when she has precisely 600 calories left for dinner, based on the planning of her day and the person that she chooses to be, one of her coworkers will invite her out for drinks.

Now, that sounds like fun, who doesn't want a little more social time in their life? A few cocktails and a few laughs. Her typical response, "Sounds like fun!" Immediately Meg's mind is split, she knows that she wants to weigh 135 pounds. She knows that she would feel amazing about herself at that number, that she would feel better, look better and be healthier, but she doesn't want the people that invited her to think that she can't go because she wants to lose weight, so she'll just drink vodka and soda when she goes out. At 90 calories each, that's no problem.

You may have experienced what happens next, a few drinks later, Meg says in her mind, "Oh well, it is too late now, let's go get pizza!" Her subconscious mind ran the program, what others think of you is more important than what you wish for yourself and the deal was done. The next day, Meg wakes up feeling bad about herself and her ditch of good days versus bad days is now a little deeper.

Remember, every day your brain is learning your preferences, ALL of your preferences, even the ones that we program in so that we can get up, look in the mirror and be unhappy or dissatisfied. Which leads me to one of the most important questions that you can ever ask yourself.

The question

Will eating this or doing this today bring me peace today AND tomorrow?
The key phrase in the question is, of course, "and tomorrow."

•*But Helena, I can't eat my number when I travel, I end up in so many fast food restaurants.*

Go in with a plan. Most calorie counts are online. A cheeseburger

Happy Meal with fries and a bottle of water equals 400 calories. Plus, you get a toy.

•*But Helena, I want people to like me.*

It is way more important to like yourself. Once you like and dare I say even love yourself, others will follow the lead.

•*But Helena, I really want chocolate cake! Fine, this may be your dinner.*

After a few days, you will need and want real food.

The choice

Every moment of every day you get to make a choice with the most advanced super computer known to man—your conscious mind.

You get to decide who it is that you are programming your subconscious mind to be. You get to choose. Each time that you make the choice for you, your brain learns that this is the preference and will play this program called your Life in Synergy, called you at peace. In the beginning the choice can seem so hard, this is because your brain is playing a different pattern. It is playing the pattern of, "I want to wake up tomorrow disliking myself."

The more you make the choice the more you will live it. Then on one fateful day, you are out with your friends and they say, let's go get pizza after cocktails and you say, "No, I am going home." The next day, you wake up having chosen a new pattern to play. Or after a stressful day at work when you would normally reach for the pint of ice cream (isn't a pint a single serving size?), instead you go home and cook yourself a real dinner because you are the most important person in your world.

Your body and your life are your choice!

Your life

Realize that as you have been going along, programming in the person you are now you have also been educating the world around you to this preference. Which means that if you are like Meg, there are probably people all around you ready to give you chocolate cake or mac and cheese at the first signs of stress.

Don't be angry at them, they are only following your plan. This is why the gang always asks Meg to join them, they know that she will say yes. If you do not put yourself first, no one else will do it for you. You have to choose your own life. Often, people will ask me what I eat each day, they want to eat exactly as I do.

I tell them 1,625. If they just copied the foods that I eat, they would be living my life not discovering their own. Yes, the last section of this book will cover some of the basic science of your different choices but you really have to learn that the choice is yours to make. You have to be responsible for you, no one else can.

You can never hear this enough.

Your love affair with you

Now is your moment to find real peace and harmony in the only place that it exists, within your heart and mind. As you find your peace, your happiness as you make the choice to have peace today and tomorrow, you set up a chain reaction of possibility.

Changing the programming in your brain can seem like a daunting task, but remember it all begins with a single step. One single change in action. There was a very popular book about a decade ago called "The Art of Possibility." In the beginning of a semester, this teacher gave each of his students an A before they even began and then allowed and encouraged them to live up to it. They not only succeeded, they exceeded his and their expectations.

Know that as you begin to make the choice for you, you have an advocate. In my mind, I have given each of you an A.

I know that you can and will be successful. I know that each of you will find your peace and happiness.

Here are some mechanics to make the transition:

1. Identify your ditch.

Only by taking an honest assessment of your life can you plan a path to success. When you are stressed, do you eat in front of the TV or grab a trashy novel and a bag of chips? Recognize your pattern and choose differently. When stress starts to mount, get up and walk. I do not care where. To the bathroom, to get a glass of water, around the block, up and down your apartment or house. Do you turn on the same show or pick the same magazine or book? Change the pattern, choose a different channel, music instead of TV, dance in your kitchen, paint. It can be paint by numbers, who cares? Toward the end of your day, send yourself a reminder about how you want to feel tomorrow.

2. Think outside of yourself.

Realize that when you are in the moment you may default to a ditch pattern that will not leave you at peace tomorrow. This is where technology really comes in handy. Set an alarm on your phone that says, "Choose to live in peace." Put up a sticky note. Find an affirmation. Take a moment to breathe. Remind yourself about your new choice and your new life.

3. Be firm in your choice.

I was recently working with a client that felt herself slipping back in to her ditch. She had recently moved out of the city so her 10,000 steps were not clear in her mind and she had fallen in to a pattern where she was putting her 2-year-old in front of herself. Skipping her walks because he was slow and complained about it. My suggestion, get him involved, teach him how to support you, know what is essential to your happiness and do not let go.

Well, it worked. She may have had to slow down, but getting those steps in is not a race.

Change your mind and change your life and then the whole world will learn from you. Your choice is not only important to you, but it is important for the whole world.

Each time you choose peace and happiness, the rest of the world learns about it and experiences it.

You are more powerful and more amazing than you can ever know.

Choose you, your peace and your love affair with you.

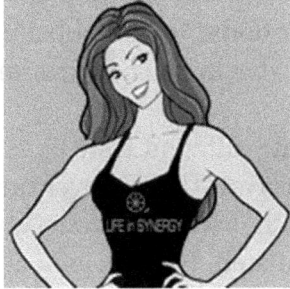

CHAPTER 10

TASTE BUD ALIGNMENT

Have you ever wondered why you have different taste buds? These little sensory gems on your tongue are there for you to experience food in multiple ways.

First, they are your early detection system along with your sense of smell to let you know if something is fresh and safe for your system. How many times have you grabbed that questionable carton of milk, taken a sniff and not been sure if it should be tossed? If there is no one else around for a second opinion, the next step is a little taste. Your taste buds have learned the taste of milk, and if that initial sip is not up to par, they send warning signals to your brain.

Yelling, Wait, stop! This will make you sick!, they are the perfect guardians.

Secondly, taste buds act as sensory agents, letting you experience the food that nourishes you on an emotional level. Think about eating your favorite food, savoring every bite. Just the thought of the taste of it stimulates the pleasure sensors in your brain. It's thanks to your taste buds that you can choose your comfort and celebration foods. Finally, your taste buds, when properly aligned, can help you regulate the foods you need to fully nourish your body. You already know how your brain is constantly evolving to survive in your environment.

Your food choices stimulate different taste buds and set your brain up with cravings for your survival. This is never more apparent than with the trifecta of wealth, which is why our sweet and salty taste buds are most often the most stimulated. But let's look at all of them in more detail.

Identifying your tastes

Your tongue comes equipped with five types of taste buds: sweet, salty, bitter, sour and umami.

Each one is designed to encourage you to eat a different type of food for optimal health. At my studio, I am constantly talking with clients about their physical alignment or engineering. Each muscle in your body is designed for a specific job and purpose. We briefly touched on this in the chapter on exercise, you overuse some muscles and under-use others, your body responds in a multitude of ways, mostly with pain and personal frustration. The same is true about your taste buds. Let's go over the alignment of each taste, what kinds of foods they are designed to encourage you to eat, and how to realign them.

Sweet

The sweet taste bud is primarily for fruit. Have you ever noticed that you crave something sweet after a meal? That is fruit's shining moment. Besides the health benefits of vitamins and nutrients found in fruit, fruit is filled with water and fiber. We are going to go into fiber in more detail a little bit later on, but basically, fiber helps you to digest your food and to slow down how quickly your stomach empties. In other words, the fiber in fruit helps you to feel full longer and to stabilize your blood sugar levels after your meals. Your body knows this; it wants to feel full and to be able to utilize the fuel you have just given it efficiently so it sends out a craving for sweet after every meal. Fruit is going to help your body digest better and act as a multi-vitamin to prevent disease and keep you healthy. Many of your anti-oxidants, which translate to anti-aging properties, are found in fruit.

Salty

The salty taste bud is there to help you maintain adequate water in your system and to help your brain and nerve functions. That's why a saline drip is pre- scribed for someone hospitalized for dehydration. Sodium (found in salt) is one of the electrolytes that I like to call the "iums:" sodium, potassium, calcium and magnesium.

All of these vital nutrients enable your body and brain to function, your muscles to contract, and your metabolism to reach its optimal levels.

Sour

The sour taste bud is for whole grains, nuts, seeds and citrus. These foods often make up the bulk of our calories, like all of the other tastes these foods are filled with health benefits, fiber and nutrients.

Bitter

Bitter is for the vegetables in your life. We often completely shut off the bitter taste bud. I cannot tell you how many people I meet who never eat any vegetables. (You are not alone!) Besides being low in calories, vegetables are high in fiber, vitamins and minerals, all of which are necessary for optimal health.

Many of the typical health problems that occur may be prevented with a few vegetables in your life. Have you ever heard someone that goes on a diet talk about how much energy they have? That is because the foods that are associated with bitter are filled with so many vitamins.

Umami

Only recently discovered, umami is for the protein in your life: the fish, the beef, the poultry. This taste can also be identified as savory. All of you who prefer to snack on cheese than on chips know what this taste is all about. This taste is about the fullness of life.

Understanding your Taste Bud Alignment®

Now that I have you thinking about those little bumps on your tongue let's dis- cuss how they end up being misaligned in the first place.

Sweet

If you have a hyperactive sweet taste bud, at some point in your life, after a meal or when you needed some quick energy, you grabbed a candy bar or cupcake instead of an apple. (If only they had those by convenience store registers.)

The first time you do this, your body observes the behavior. The second time, your body starts to pay attention. After a few days, your body learns that this is your preference. At this point, your body preempts your future choice by giving you a craving for the cookie or candy instead, and a pattern emerges.

Your body thinks that whatever you are feeding it is for its best interest. It replaces its need for fruit for a need for a cookie. Have you ever noticed how little kids love fruit? They have not had a chance to teach their taste buds something new, so the fruit is right on! How do you correct this?

Have a piece of fruit after every meal. Not juice, just fruit. The first change that you are going to notice is how filling it will be, and how much better you will feel, after lunch especially. The fruit will give you a quick burst of energy while slowing down how quickly the rest of your meal gets digested. Translation: you will feel energized by your lunch instead of craving a nap. (Bonus: You'll save a bundle by not having to pick up an afternoon coffee every day.) You will feel energized all afternoon because the fiber in the fruit keeps your blood sugar levels more even.

100

Instead of a quick high followed by a quick low, you will be fully fueled. This is the key to leading an active life. You need to have the constant supply of energy to keep going.

• *But Helena, what about all of those diets that tell me that fruit is evil?*

In case you cannot feel my eyes rolling right now, they are. No one ever lost their balance by eating fruit. Fruit is nature's candy, the sweetness of life. As you reintroduce it in to your life, you will see first-hand how amazing it is. Health benefits of a strawberry include preventing heart disease, Alzheimer's and cancer. They are anti-inflammatory, have a low glycemic index, and have more nutrients than you even know. Ellegic acid anyone? Pantothenic acid, vitamin K, manganese? You will not see any of these things in a candy bar. You also won't find the group of greatest hits like vitamin C, potassium and fiber. All this from a strawberry. Sounds like a miracle drug, doesn't it? This is all for less than 50 calories per cup. (That equals the caloric content of five peanut M&M's—and who can ever have just five?) If you're really craving sweet, try a cup of strawber- ries with a packet of raw sugar on top.

Total calories...wait for it...63!

There is another culprit - the artificial sweetener

I remember sitting in the studio one afternoon when my student Judy walked in the door. She had been doing the online version of my program, receiving one lesson a day for 30 days. This way you can really digest (pun intended) each lesson before moving on to the next. Judy was always excited; she was learning how to eat, she was happy, and she was not stressing about every bite that she took. Then she got to the chapter about artificial sweeteners. That day, she walked in and was totally freaking out, arms crossed, nervous and anxious.

She was ready to dispute the rule.

I told her the same thing I'll tell your skeptical mind. First, think back to being a little kid after having some sugar, or even some berries, running around like crazy. That's the sugar high. As a child, your body learns that sweet means energy. Now in come the artificial sweeteners, often

ten to 100 times sweeter than sugar, but with zero calories which means no energy or sustenance for your body. Remember, your body learned that sweet means energy, and suddenly it is experiencing super sweet and no energy because there are no calories in artifi- cial sweeteners.

This confuses your body to no end, and it starts to wonder if it needs any more energy. It remedies this by sending out a hunger signal. It says to your brain, "Listen we are having a malfunction down here, I received the sweet thing that you sent, but right now, I've got nothing! Can you send something else please? I mean it, this is a crisis. Send me more energy!" Who knew that your body was so excitable? Here is the reality: there are 17 calories in a packet of sugar. That's not the culprit of your diet failing, but this overcompensation from artificial sweeteners could be.

Very reluctantly, Judy took the artificial sweetener out of her life. (And this was a woman who had people ship it to her for a year when she lived in Japan.) Judy is now sweetener-free. She uses a little cinnamon in her coffee instead. (Try it, you will love it and cinnamon is great for your heart.) Her skin looks amazing and she feels in control of her life.
In addition to having no calories, artificial sweeteners also completely mess up your taste buds because they are super sweet, making fruit nev- er sweet enough to satisfy. Remember, your body is learning. It is your responsibility to teach and care for it.

One of my clients lost 40 pounds last year. The only change we made in her eating? No more diet drinks. Once she replaced them with water, she was less hungry, so she consumed fewer calories in total and lost the weight. Those drinks have the same number of calories as water, but the stuff from your tap can do far less damage to your body.

The sweet taste bud is usually one of the most misaligned, but it's your responsibility to change it. Changing your patterns is really about com- mitting to yourself, your life, your well-being and your ultimate happi- ness and peace. All this can be achieved by choosing an orange over the cookie, a little cinnamon over the artificial sweetener.

•*But Helena, I LOVE chocolate…*

A Life in Synergy is a life in balance. If you love chocolate or cake or candy, make a plan for it. Train your body to eat more fruit, but plan your calories for the treats that feed your being. Realize also that we all have pity party days. Em- brace it! Grab the party hat, the noisemaker and the chocolate cake, and relax. I once ate my entire 1,625 calories in cake and champagne. Trust me, after one day of that, all you want is a salad. This is really a Life in Synergy.

Salty

When you are dehydrated, your body will naturally crave salty foods to help you retain as much water as possible. The problem with a mis- aligned salty taste bud is that increased sodium intake can lead to high blood pressure which can, in turn, lead to heart disease. In addition, as your body takes in sodium, it rejects potassium, creating another imbal- ance. This can all be remedied by just drink- ing more water.

For every pound that you weigh, you need half an ounce of water. So if you weigh 140 pounds, drink 70 ounces of water today and get your salty taste bud back in to alignment. Just to remind you of the other benefits of water: better digestion, better comprehension, better sleep habits, less muscle cramping, increased energy, and an overall more efficient you. How did our diets become the salt lick that they are today? Salt is nature's preservative, so if you are a food manufacturer and you want your food to last longer so that you do not have to factor in spoil- age costs, you add salt.

It is how many of our ancestors survived through the winter, preserving meats and vegetables. Almost every time that you eat something out of a bag or a box, it has added sodium in it. How much of this essential nu- trient do you need? The American Heart Association recommends that you have 1,000 mg per 1,000 calories of food. Ideally, I would have 1,625 mg of sodium per day. Trust me, on that pizza therapy day, I am blowing that number out of the water. But on a regular day-to-day basis, I often do not get enough, which has contributed to some low blood pressure and the occasional headache.

I know when I'm low on sodium because suddenly I start craving olives. This is my active salty taste bud in action, which now as I think about it may have been how pizza therapy started in the first place. As I take the time to look at myself, I now realize that I really crave pizza therapy on my low sodium weeks and often blow it off when I have been eating a more balanced diet during the week. This is the best part about learning about yourself. There is always something new to discover.

•*But Helena, I don't want to look at how much sodium something has.*

Creating your own Life in Synergy is so exciting. Each day you get to learn something new about yourself. Take the time to care for the most important person in your world: you. The great part, it is the 21st century. Information is at your fingertips.

Learn about you.

Add your ideal sodium intake to your number and spend a week carefully mon- itoring it so that you can feel the balance. You will be amazed at how unbeliev- able your body will feel when it is balanced. You'll have energy from morning to night. I would be remiss if I did not mention the other extreme of salty, over hydrating. I recently had a client who was constantly craving salt.

As we talked about her eating and drinking habits I discovered that she was over hydrating, drinking more than a gallon of water a day. Her body was constantly craving salt because she was depleting her body of all of her electrolytes, literally flushing her essential nutrients right out of her system. A Life in Synergy is a life of balance, know what is right for you. This is really the goal—for each of us to find our personal balance, what makes our bodies, minds and spirits soar. Do not look to someone else for his or her answer; you have to find your own to really understand your ideal.

Sour

Like its bitter counterparts, often this taste bud is under-utilized and under-developed, or it has been processed out of your taste awareness.

To learn about this taste bud, try to eat sour foods that look very similar to their original form:

- whole grain bread vs. white bread
- a grapefruit vs. grapefruit juice
- brown rice vs. white rice
- whole milk yogurts vs. the corn syrup sweetened low-fat version
- real peanut butter vs. the sweetened version

You are going to see these foods pop up in every category as we progress through the book. If you want to reduce your risk of cancer, digestive issues and chronic disease, then your diet needs to have some sour aspects. Notice how we have altered the food in this taste category to make them a part of our overactive sweet taste. In each of the examples above, the original food has been processed down and sugar has been added.

This does two things: it makes these taste buds inactive and it puts your sweet taste buds into overdrive. If you teach your sour taste bud that it should not work, and that sweet is the preference, you will crave more sweetness each day until a cookie addiction is born. But now you know better than to give into that craving. It's just your sweet taste buds over-stimulated, while the rest of your taste buds are not doing their jobs.

Think about your taste buds as a small division of a company. The company works at peak performance when everyone knows their jobs and executes them efficiently. In the taste bud division, the salty and sweet workers are working all the time, while the rest of the workers (here's looking at you bitter and sour) get to come in late and take long breaks. Now, it is easy to just blame them for not doing their job, but what about the CEO? Did she fully explain their duties? Years ago, their assignments (real food) were everywhere, readily available to the company.

Now, in modern America, the CEO has to work a little harder to get these contracts, but that is the CEO's job. Your job as the CEO of your body is to give bitter and sour more work so that sweet and salty can take a much-needed vacation. Take the time to teach sour its job so it will do it all on its own. It needs your encouragement.

Here are a few ways to incorporate sour:

- Add a few nuts or seeds to your diet each day. Use them sparingly because these nutrition powerhouses are also heavy on calories. Just sprinkle a few on top of a salad or add them to real yogurt.

- Try a slice of grainy bread, the nuttier looking, the better. I like mine toasted with a little butter.

- Skip the juice and have half a grapefruit. Get yourself a grapefruit spoon and try to scoop out a whole section—there is nothing more satisfying.

- Instead of having white rice with your dinner, try a brown or even a nuttier native version.

The great thing about all of these changes is that you are not only taking the time to educate your sour taste buds, but you are also adding a ton of health-promot- ing fiber into your life. This will not only make you feel better, it will make you feel full longer. If you are hungry all the time, this is your ticket to health and fullness.

Bitter

Like sour, the bitter taste buds get almost turned off from not being used fre- quently enough, which is why many people hate vegetables. That's why it's best to introduce one vegetable serving at a time. Add a little fat at first to dull the taste and then gradually decrease the fat on the top so that you can fully appreciate this rich taste. As you introduce the bitter taste, not to mention all of those vitamins, your body will quickly adjust and turn on the bitter cravings. Yes, you will suddenly want veggies with your meal (and we're not talking carrot cake).

That is why we gradually increase the amount of vegetables and fruit over the 21 days of the Trifecta of Health.

A Life in Synergy is a life of health and variety.

Instead of thinking about what you cannot have, think about what you need for the care and maintenance of your body. I was working with a client who was having a really hard time getting her veggies in every day, so we made a plan: lunch is veggie hour. Every day at lunch, she has either a salad or vegetable soup. She piles all kinds of things in to her salad, every veggie on the bar, and then tops it with a little blue cheese dressing.

Yummy! She would have three cups of vegetables (150 calories), 2 tablespoons of blue cheese dressing (180 calories) and either a hard-boiled egg, some nuts, or a quarter cup of seeds (with each of these proteins coming in at 75-80 calories). Don't have a calculator on hand? Allow me.

That grand total for that mound of food is between 405 and 410 calories. Eating a big salad is civilized, enjoyable and relaxing (which is fitting because you de- serve only the best mealtime experience). On the days that client chooses soup instead, we add a whole grain roll with butter, which makes the meal last longer and be more satisfying. If it's a soup day, count between 180 and 300 calories for 16 ounces of soup, 140 calories for two slices of whole grain bread, and 60 calo- ries for two teaspoons of butter. That total can range from 380 to 500 calories.

The most important part about these small changes is that this client feels amaz- ing, she is getting her veggies in every day and she has even started craving some at dinner. All we had to do was help the CEO (her brain) come up with a plan to teach the bitter taste bud its job.

Umami

This taste is about the fullness of life and it often gets misaligned when it is used to feed emotions as well as hunger. An overactive Umami or savory taste bud is often brought back to an alignment with an activity other than eating.

Try something savory for your soul, like:

- Listening to music.

- Going for a walk.

- Dancing.

- Arranging Flowers.

- Reading.

- Playing a video game.

Fill this taste bud with the love for your life.

As with all of the other tastes, keep it simple to truly appreciate the subtleties in the flavor. We often mask this flavor, when you eat a burger you have masked the flavor of the meat with cheese, ketchup, bread, etc.

The toppings we add to our umami taste are often from that overdeveloped duo of sweet and salty.

Simplify and explore the savory side of your life.

Recognizing your overdeveloped buds

What foods do you crave?

If you are having a bad day or are ready to celebrate, do you reach for the choc- olate, the chips or the cheese? (Interesting how it's probably the same food, isn't it?) Utilizing the plan for the trifecta of health will often help you better align your tastes and begin to develop craving for salads, but sometimes we all need to take a second look.

Keeping a food journal for a week can be one of the most eye-opening exercises. Not only will you see how your taste buds are influencing your choices, but you will also be able to see your patterns. At the beginning of the book, you may have looked at the three types and put your self in the thinker category, but after writing a food journal you may notice that your choices are very different on the weekends.

Maybe you are a commuter. Perhaps you never crave bitter foods but you drink five cups of coffee each day. After a few cups, your bitter taste feels as though its job is done.

Making a plan for balance

A journal that starts with food can lead to endless self-discoveries.

Writing down your choices as well as your emotions, your thoughts and your feelings can better help you understand yourself. I know that often when I write, I am shocked at what I discover.

•What is it that you really want?

•Is it the cookie, or is it a moment of peace?

•Is it the chips, or is it a quiet mind? Is it the cheese, or is it a feeling of satisfaction?

•Food and tastes can seem like an easy fix in the moment, but how will you feel tomorrow?

A Life in Synergy is not a life of perfection, but a life of peace, health and happiness that brings you beyond perfection to fulfillment.

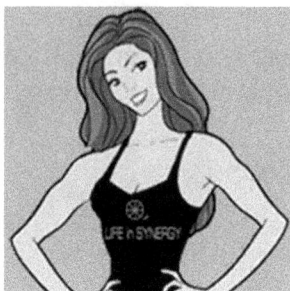

CHAPTER 11

FIBER - THE WORKOUT FOR YOUR INSIDES

Here's a fun fact: The human body has between 25 and 28 feet of intestines, if you were to stretch them from end to end.

That is a long way for your food to have to travel everyday.

Just like the muscle that moves you to take a walk, your intestines are filled with muscles that move your food through all 20-something feet on the inside. Everything that you eat is pushed through your system of intestines with a muscle contraction called a peristaltic movement, the rhythm of digestion.

The small intestine is there to help you digest and absorb the nutrients of your food, and the large intestine absorbs water, sodium and other trace elements. (Here's another reminder of the importance of water: In the digestive process, it helps your food move more easily through the first 20 feet.) In order for all of this to happen as efficiently as possible, you have to maintain the strength, endurance and capability of these all-important muscles.

Like all muscles, you either use them or lose them. It is your job to keep them at their physical peak, and figure out the most effective workout. (Thankfully for your tummy, no dumbbells are involved.)

Fiber: The overview

Fiber is the workout for your insides and is essential for intestinal health.

No wonder there are so many commercials on every day for fiber supplements, fiber added to other foods and fiber to keep you regular. There is no need for supplements though (unless your doctor has prescribed them). That same fiber those commercials are trying to sell you is found in all of your fruits, vegetables, whole grains, nuts and seeds. These foods are not only powerhouses of nutrients, but they are also nature's workout for your insides, helping to keep them in shape so they can work effectively.

This is why fiber rich foods can be, well, a workout on your system as you add them into your diet. Be sure to add them gradually over a month (or risk spending a bit too much time "powdering your nose" at work). You would not start a new workout routine by running a marathon. Your leg muscles would get fatigued and stressed, and they would be unable to complete the workout. Not only that, but how often have you gone to a killer workout and then not gone back for a month or two? The same holds true for your insides. You need to gradually increase your fiber intake to get your insides back in shape.

Here is the important part: Just like aligning your taste buds so that your body will begin to crave different tastes and foods, your insides will begin to crave a good workout. You will find yourself wanting a salad, some fruit or whole grain bread, nuts and seeds. Every single part of your body has a job to do. Your body wants to be active, it is just waiting for an explanation and some training to get the job done.

In order to understand fiber, we need to understand what happened to it in our regular diet. Where did it all disappear to? It was mostly processed out to make eating more food easier and to make things last longer on the shelf. A piece of fruit will last about a week at the grocery store, but bottled juice can sit on a shelf for a year. This is processing. Any time you change your food from its original form, you have processed it in some way. As whole grains are ground down, fruit is turned into juice, your food is able to slide through your intestines without needing to be broken down and pushed through.

The muscles in your intestines get out of shape and the food without fiber just slips through your body more easily, leaving your body to constantly ask you for more.

At some point your body, or even your ancestor's body, processed real food, so your genetic memory knows how long it takes to digest something. When something just slides through, your body gets confused and it is not really sure if it had enough. Think about if you had to walk 10 miles to the mall to go shopping. You would limit your shopping, knowing you would have to lug those purchases all the way home afterward.

Obviously you still need a cute outfit and new shoes, but you would not go on a shopping spree. You would choose just the perfect things for you because your body can only do so much carrying and walking. There is a natural limit that you understand. Instead, we zip to the mall in our cars with plenty of room for those shopping bags. Instead of picking one great outfit, we know that we can have many. How many times have you purchased the perfect shirt only to come home and realize that you have five others just like it? Then, that perfect shirt gets shoved in to the over-crowded closet.

This is what has happened to our processed food. The processing made getting and keeping our food easier, so we keep on getting more and more. None of it makes us feel or look better, and our bodies end up cluttered. As you begin to be more selective, you will get added benefits just like the compliments you get on that great outfit. Let's talk about those benefits of fiber.

The added benefits of fiber

• Reduced risk for most disease

•Steadier blood sugar levels

•Lower LDL (bad) cholesterol

• Prevention of some cancers

•Feeling full longer

•Keeps you clean, this is nature's detox

The last one is probably my favorite. Have you heard all of those ads for detox products, or people talking about toxins in your system? Eat an orange instead. They are nature's yummy, nutrient- and vitamin-filled detoxifier. How much fiber you need depends on how many calories you eat each day.

The standard recommendation is 14 grams for each 1,000 calories you eat, so I need approximately 22 grams per day.

That is a couple of pieces of fruit, a few servings of vegetables and a few pieces of whole grain bread. It's not as complicated as they make it seem on TV. It really comes down to getting 50 percent of your calories from natural carbohydrates like fruits, veggies and whole grains.

Fiber comes in two forms: insoluble and soluble.

Insoluble-your backhoe

Just like it sounds, insoluble fiber does not dissolve or change in your system.

It goes out the same way that it goes in. (Think of corn.) This type of fiber moves bulk through your system.

Insoluble fiber is the heavy lifter, the resistance training for your insides.

It is like the backhoe for your intestines, pushing the bulk. This requires that your intes- tines stay in shape to push this heavy lifter through. Besides being a great work- out, insoluble fiber also controls the pH (acidity) in your intestines, pH diets are the latest craze. To maintain an ideal pH in your system, you just need to get good sources of insoluble fiber in to your diet on most days. Start by eating the skin of the apple and you'll be on your way.

Insoluble fiber also removes toxic waste from the colon and helps in the preven- tion of colon cancer.

Are you sick of everyone talking about toxins? I know I am. Well, here is nature's built in detox that you can do every day for a toxin-free life.

Fruit skins, root vegetables, whole wheat, whole grains, seeds and nuts are all sources. Eat the skin of your baked potato, have your sandwich on whole grain bread, eat the apple with the skin and throw a few nuts and seeds on your salad at lunch.

Soluble-Daily Detox

Soluble fiber dissolves in the stomach and becomes sort of like tapioca.

This acts like a super cleansing gel for your intestines, getting into every nook and cranny for a thorough detox. In addition to lowering cho- lesterol by binding with fatty acids, this fiber prolongs the time it takes for your stomach to empty, meaning you feel full for much longer. This slower emptying equates to slower absorption of sugar into your blood stream. That's why you do not get the same kind of sugar rush or high with an orange that you would get with a candy bar; the orange is filled with soluble fiber. Soluble fiber helps you to stay even and energized instead of falling in to the yo-yo cycle often associated with other simple carbohydrates.

This fiber is found in oats, nuts, dried beans, barley, flax seed, oranges, apples and carrots, just to name a few of my favorites. This is one of my favorite show-and-tell moments in my nutrition lectures. I love showing people how Chia seeds (yes, just like the ones on the pet) dissolve and expand in water. A little tiny seed becomes a gelatinous mass sort of like tapioca.

This is what happens to soluble fiber in your stomach and intestines, except that it is combining with fatty acids, also known as cholesterol. This healthy tapioca then goes through every nook and cranny of your 20 plus feet of intestines and cleans them out. Have some beans at your next barbecue, and at the end of the day be ready to be energized, thoroughly clean and detoxed.

Finding a source

Are you beginning to see a pattern emerge?

When you choose a food that your brain recognizes, it satisfies your taste buds and helps them to stay in balance. That may be a part of your trifecta of health— you are often picking a food that will keep your insides in shape, prevent disease and keep you even and fueled throughout your day.

Often this food will automatically self-regulate as far as serving size, so you don't have to worry or spend time thinking about how much you have had. The foods that keep your body healthy also keep your mind healthy. Not only do they provide key nutrients and vitamins but they also reduce the stress and thinking about your body, your weight, your health and eating your number. Choosing
a vegetable is not a hardship, it is a testament to how much you love and care about yourself.

It is a means to a better body, better skin, looking and feeling hotter and giving yourself the very best.

This is a Life in Synergy. Change your mind about fiber-rich foods not because you are forced to eat something, but because you deserve the best life, because you deserve to be in love with yourself and your body, because you deserve to feel great and energized to live a full and happy life. So much of how we feel about certain foods is just a pattern. Instead of living, we are constantly reacting. Teaching our minds and bodies to be constantly worried and stressed instead of learning to fully enjoy and embrace our lives. Stop for a moment and really think about it.

Pick foods that are real. Have a piece of fruit at the end of your meals. Detox ev- ery day. Get in your three servings of veggies and energize your life. Throw a few nuts and seeds on top of the salad to put your body and mind in to hyper drive. Toast a beautiful piece of nutty whole grain bread and bring your sandwich to a whole new level of excellence.

Once you have fueled yourself, the glass of wine or piece of cake will taste that much better, you will appreciate it that much more and you will wake up tomor- row in love with the most important person in your life... you!

Having a plan

Having said all of that, sometimes it is best just to have a plan. Look at your food journal and see where you are having trouble getting in your fiber and trifecta of health. It may be a simple substitution that makes all of the difference.

Do you eat a muffin in the morning? Try some oatmeal. I like mine with brown sugar and raisins.

Do you have a sandwich at lunch? Try a salad or vegetable soup.

Do you crave a cookie after your meal? Try some sliced apples with cin- namon and sugar on them instead.

Don't do these things because you need to punish yourself, but because you deserve the absolute best in life.

Take the time to learn about you and your patterns.

You are so interesting.

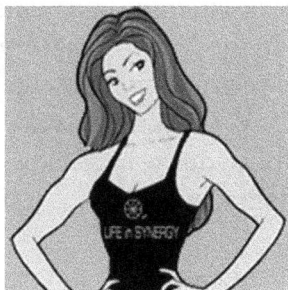

CHAPTER 12

INFLAMMATION AND HEALTH

We all have a pair; those shoes we just had to have, even if they were a half size too small and a few inches too high. And those six straps? Well, that's the style this fall, right? We wear them even if they make our feet hurt, because they make our minds feel great.

We feel sexy, unstoppable and, most importantly, confident. But the blisters start to appear before we've even made it to dinner. Sometimes, no matter how great our minds feel, our bodies fight back.

Clearly these are not the healthiest option, but essential in our lives. The same goes for what you eat. Those high processed foods, saturated in sugar and trans fats, can make you feel better after a hard day at work, but eating too much of them can lead to health issues and disease. If you can get it from a drive-through window, it is probably an inflammatory food. If we used food solely for fuel, we could easily drop these meals from our diets. But we have learned to feed our physical body, as well as our minds. (That double cheeseburger brings you back to summer vacation; those chicken fingers are the ones your favorite babysitter used to serve.)

Food is our source of energy, vitamins, nutrients and life. A Life in Synergy includes pleasure from food. Inflammatory foods are filled with the Trifecta of Wealth. When we are starving mentally and emotionally, we tend to turn to these foods. We look to the cake and ice cream to soothe our emotions, it is a subconscious way of showing ourselves that we are deserving of wealth, strength and power.

The key is understanding and balance. If not, the physical part of our being gets overwhelmed and abused by this behavior and we end up out of balance and not in optimal health. That then taxes our emotional and mental parts of our being, and before you know it you have purchased a ticket on the merry-go-round of unhappiness and disease. (And wasn't that pint of ice cream supposed to be the solution?) I am here to guide you to the exit off of this ride. It is important to have a plan to not only feed our physical bodies but one for our emotional and mental bodies as well, especially when it comes to balancing your inflammatory food intake.

Feeding your mental and emotional bodies

We have all experienced mental exhaustion.

You spent the entire day in your office, never moving from your chair, glued to your desk and you are so tired you can barely move. You can barely keep your eyes open, which doesn't make sense and you know it. You didn't run a marathon, you weren't swimming laps in the pool. You sat all day. This is mental exhaustion. Ordering a pizza seems so much easier than actually figuring out what to cook that night. A little salt, fat and sugar will be fast, easy and comforting.

But will it?

Here's what's really going on:

First, remember, you are probably dehydrated. Your brain is 85 percent water, more than any other part of your body. Two things happen in an office: the air system circulates dry air, and you get too consumed by your work to remem- ber to sip from that water bottle. If you do not give your body water, it will ask for food to solve this important problem and before you even realize what is happening you are at the vending machine or picking up an extra cup of coffee, exceeding your chemical limit for the day along with a cookie or brownie.

Second, you are probably stuck on the "to-do ride" in this amusement park of horrors. It's like getting stuck in that "why treadmill" with a toddler, where you can never have enough answers to their endless stream of questions. This happens with our own brains. You are running through the same problem or to do list over and over again. It can feel like there is a skipping record in your head. Thinkers and Decorators can especially get stuck in this mode, either obsessing about it or trying to perfect everything. All of this over thinking takes energy, and your brain starts to get tired.

It knows that when the rest of your body is tired, food breaks down to energy so it sends out a craving: I'm stressed, feed me, medicate me, buy me a cocktail, buy me another cocktail, and, oh yeah, feed me!

Recognizing your brain fatigue is key, and understanding how to refuel it is essential. First drink some water, then try a quick walk. Walking oxygenates your brain, and it's like putting your brain on added life sup- port. Even two minutes of walking in place will make a difference. Fol- low this by physically removing the "to do" thoughts from your brain. Write them down, send your self a text (but not while driving, please) or shoot yourself an e-mail, and then sing a song. Yes, that's what I said, sing a song. It can be in your head, or even a soft hum.

Think of the last time you sang at the top of your lungs. Were you wor- rying about your problems or thinking about going grocery shopping and doing laundry? Of course not. Your brain needs rest, relaxation and a little exercise every day, just like your body.

How are you treating your brain?

• Are you constantly working it out without any rest?

• Are you going from a sprint to a crash?

• Are you forcing it to run endlessly on a treadmill, thinking about the never-ending to do list?

• Are you constantly thinking about what's going to happen next?

• Are you spending time thinking about what others are thinking about?

These habits become self-sustaining, which can be taxing and exhausting.

Your brain is probably in need of some balance and some rest. Here are a few ways that I like to help my mental body stay in shape:

• I read two books at a time: an easy, fun read and something that will challenge my brain. It keeps my mind flexible and in shape.

• When a work issue pops into my head, I write it on my to do list, even if it has woken me up at 2 a.m.

• I have quiet time every morning, allowing my brain to wander.

• I enjoy Sudoku puzzles, and will do them without stressing whenever I find them in a paper or magazine.

• When work is stressful and I find myself being unproductive, I go for a walk and sing in my head (OK, sometimes out loud).

• I shut my phone off and go off the grid once I get home.

• If I know that I am going to have a stressful week, I plan my meals ahead of time, factoring in dessert for the week in my number.

By recognizing your mind, you can learn to care and feed it just like you have your physical body.

Your emotional body is different from your mental one.

This is your area of celebration and sadness: your heart. Scientists have found that a cluster of nerve cells around your heart send signals to your brain, instead of visa versa. In other words, sometimes your heart is doing your thinking and telling your brain and your body how to react. There is a reason that both a birthday and a break up often involve chocolate cake and ice cream. Your emo- tional body is asking to be fed.

Just like your physical and mental body, this part of you needs to be recognized and nourished.

Let's start with recognition. What are you feeling?

• What is the first feeling you have when you wake up?

• How do you feel on your way to work?

• What feelings do you have when you talk to your friends?

• How do you decide when you are deciding what to eat?

• How do you feel before you go to sleep?

By taking the time to look at what you are feeling, you will be better able to feed this part of you. Are you blocking feelings or trying to manage them with food? Are your emotions preventing you from succeeding? Or are you blocking your emotions, going through your daily routines without feeling?

The simplest way to transform your emotional self and begin to feed it so that it feels full and nourished is with gratitude and breathing. Each morning when you get up begin your day with five deep breaths. Inhale for five counts, pause and hold your breath for five counts. Exhale for five counts, then pause for five counts before you begin again. The act of focused breathing calms your heart. Now think about one thing that you are grateful for.

It does not matter what it is: You have a new top, your coffee is already made thanks to the self-timer, you have a lunch date with a friend. It does not matter what you are grateful for, just that you are feeling that emotion.

Gratitude is nourishment for your emotional being. Even when you experience something difficult, you can find gratitude for what it teaches you about your- self. When I was a child, I was physically and sexually abused and left without a support system to fend for myself. This is not an experience that I would wish on anyone. But as I have gotten older, I often look to those experiences to find my gratitude. I am so thankful for what I have learned about my strength and capability.

I am so grateful that those experiences have led me to be an advocate for women and to help them find happiness and peace in their lives. I am so grateful that as I became an adult, having lived through trauma, I was not afraid of what people may think of me. I find it helpful to start with a list to get your gratitude engine in motion. List 10 things, big or small, that you are grateful for.

Each time you start to feel your emotional being in need of the richness of life, feed it with gratitude exercises and breathing before you reach for the cookie. If there is a need for added celebration at that moment, you will be in a better place to assess the situation and choose if inflammatory foods really fit the bill or not.

Remember, you are the most amazing, fabulous, interesting, exciting person in your life.

You deserve the best nourishment and health, physically, mentally and emotionally.

Nature's aspirin

Now that we have a more clear understanding about why we reach for inflammatory foods, what is the alternative? Which foods act to actively prevent disease from happening in our bodies?

Aspirin, ibuprofen and naproxen sodium work on your body because they are anti-inflammatory. They decrease inflammation to help us get rid of muscle aches, arthritis pain and headaches. You can have these same health-building effects at every meal just by including anti-inflammatory foods.

Why should that matter to you? Because besides the common ailments listed above, most disease has been directly linked to inflammation in your body. Look at these foods as the requirements for proper engine maintenance of your human vehicle and as a daily massage for your whole body.

Omega-3 fatty acids are the wonder food, more than any other supplement. Find it in walnuts, pumpkin seeds, cold water fish like salmon and trout, flax seed and, my favorite, chia seed. Chia seed is a super food, filled with fiber, ome- ga-3s and energy. I put a tablespoon in my yogurts and smoothies.

Other anti-inflammatory foods are olive oil, rice bran, grape seeds, whole grains, leafy green vegetables and colorful fruits, berries and cherries.

The balancing act

None of this has to be complicated.

•Each day, eat your trifecta of health and drink the correct amount of water.

•Pick foods that could have been produced on your grandmother's farm.

•Eat the number of calories to sustain the person that you want to be.

•Choose your treats, alcohol and processed fun foods because they are a bonus, not because you have beaten yourself up mentally and emotionally.

This is really living a Life in Synergy.

Understanding how important and amazing you are and nourishing yourself physically, mentally and emotionally.

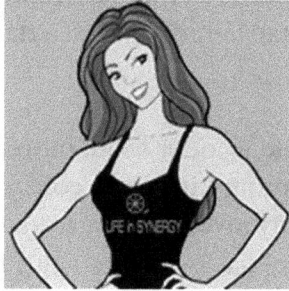

Chapter 13

Reading Labels and other
Interesting Facts

If you need a topic to really dig in to, Nutrition is it.

I spent the last five weeks researching the health benefits of herbs. Those flavor adders are not just there to make your plate look pretty, they are filled with Vitamins, anti-inflammatory and anti-bacterial (yes just like the hand sanitizer) properties.

There are so many nutrients and compounds in our food to promote health and decrease our chance of getting disease. A few weeks ago I learned quite a bit about Quercitin, a flavonoid found in many of our foods that might have anti-viral properties.

This chapter is here to pique your interest in some of the basics.

Reading labels

So what should you be looking for on a label? First, find the ingredients.

Here are some helpful hints:

• If you cannot pronounce it, put it back!

• Corn syrup, drop it!

• Artificial sweeteners, move on!

After the ingredients pass the test, find calories and serving size. Note that there is a difference.

Look at the label of a bottle of soda. Often it will say something like 120 calories. We think not bad, right? But then under serving size it will tell you that the bottle contains 2.5 servings. This means that to really understand how many calories it has, you need to multiply these numbers. Are you going to make that bottle last over the next 2.5 days? Of course not, so really that bottle of soda has 120 x 2.5 = 300 calories.

A 145 lb. moderately active woman needs approximately 1,800 calories a day to maintain her body weight. That would be one sixth of all of her calories from that one drink. If she had two bottles of soda, that is a third of all of the calories she would need in a day.

The nice thing about fruits and vegetables is that so many of them come prepackaged in a single serving size and are usually only about 50 calories a serving.

No advanced label reading required! A Life in Synergy is a life of awareness.

But back to your calories, have you ever tried to teach a small child to say please and thank you? If you have, you realize that it is a long-term process that requires consistency. Your body is absolutely no different. To really teach your body who you want to be, to never have to teach it again, to learn to be full at your caloric requirement and easily maintain your ideal weight, you must be consistent.

Put your work in at the beginning and you'll never have to work again. Your calories are your calories, they can be from fruits and vegetables, which I am sure you are learning to crave and love, or they can be from ice cream (remember the client that went on the margarita vacation?) They are just life-sustaining calories. Pick the optimal ones because you deserve the best, but pick the same amount every day to get off the switch back road and to get on the road that is your Life in Synergy.

Understanding your "iums"

It's all in the muscle!

Did you know that you burn calories by burning oxygen in your muscles?

The key to a healthy metabolism is healthy muscles. The more efficient your muscles are in contracting, the more calories you will burn every minute of every day. My goal is to burn the maximum amount of calories while sleeping. How do you keep your muscles healthy? With your iums, also known as your electrolytes.

What are your primary electrolytes?

Calcium is the most abundant mineral in your body. In addition to being necessary for muscle contraction, it also helps with your hormones, your blood vessels and obviously your teeth and bones.

Good sources of calcium include: dairy, broccoli, oranges, tofu, salmon and molasses.

Magnesium is important for muscle and nerve contraction as well as hundreds of other essential functions of the body. This mineral has also been shown to help with hypertension, diabetes and heart function.

Good sources of magnesium include: pumpkin, halibut, nuts, quinoa and spinach.

Potassium is important for muscle and nerve contraction in the body.

Good sources of potassium include: sweet potato, yogurt, bananas and clams.

Sodium is essential for pumping water into your cells, but is also the most over-consumed electrolyte in the American diet.

You need at least 500 mg a day but should not exceed 2,400. (Some Americans get more than 5,000, which can lead to hypertension.)

Good sources of sodium include: Well, I am not even going to go there.

Please note, though, if you eat mostly fresh foods and drink a lot of water, you do need sodium in your diet.

Drinking too much water and not having any sodium can lead to hypoatremia, a dangerous condition.

Vitamins

There are both water soluble and fat soluble vitamins.

The B and C vitamins are water soluble because they dissolve in the water in our bodies, so when you go to the restroom you will pass any excess of these. Vitamins A, D, E and K are fat soluble because your body stores these vitamins in your fat cells and liver and does not eliminate excess amounts of these vitamins, even if you have too much.

Vitamin A

Vitamin A comes in two forms: retinol and beta-carotene. Retinol is the animal form of vitamin A and good sources of it include eggs, liver and dairy products. Vitamin A only occurs naturally in whole milk. Reducing the fat in milk strips it of this essential vitamin, making it necessary to add a synthetic version. Beta-carotene is an organic compound and powerful anti-oxidant that turns into vitamin A in your body. Beta-carotene is found in foods with bright colors, like sweet potatoes as well as carrots, colorful peppers and apricots. Think color on your plate.

Vitamin A has many health benefits such as healthy vision and beautiful skin.

Vitamin B

There are 8 B vitamins in total, from B1 to B12. These used to be thought of as one vitamin, but research has shown that they are each distinct.

B1 is thiamin, B2 is riboflavin, B3 is niacin, B5 is pantothenic acid, B6 is pyridoxine, B7 is biotin, B9 is folic acid and B12 is, well, usually called B12. The B vitamins are essential for cell growth and development, especially for red blood cells. They are found in legumes and most sources of protein.

Vitamin C

Vitamin C is great for your immune system, but oranges aren't the only source. Strawberries, cantaloupe, papaya, broccoli, green peppers and brussels sprouts are a few examples. Vitamin C is a powerful anti-oxidant, which helps prevent aging. (Hallelujah!) With the added benefit that many of the foods high in vitamin C are also high in soluble fiber, nature's daily detox.

Vitamin D

Vitamin D is often called the "sunshine vitamin" because this vitamin is obtained primarily from exposure to sunlight. Small amounts of vitamin D can be found in fatty fish (sardines, mackerel, salmon), eggs and fortified dairy products. Vitamin D plays a major role in the building and maintenance of healthy bones and teeth due to its effect on calcium and phosphorus.

Vitamin E

Vitamin E is an antioxidant and it also protects red blood cells and cell membranes from damage. Vitamin E can be found in seeds, nuts, beans and green leafy vegetables.

Vitamin K

Not as commonly discussed as some of the other vitamins, vitamin K plays a key role in the body. The primary role of vitamin K is the formation of blood clotting substances. Research also suggests that this vitamin may help in the maintenance of healthy bones. The best sources of vitamin K are dark greens such as kale, collard greens and spinach.

A Life in Synergy is a life of balance

Now as you look at the foods that contain your electrolytes and vitamins, did you notice that you had seen them before? Remember the lessons on fiber and anti-inflammatory foods.

When trying to take care of your body, choosing these simple, whole ingredients in your daily diet help you to achieve multiple results:

• Reduce disease-causing inflammation.

• Improve the health of your insides and give your intestines a much needed daily workout.

• Detox

• Reduce your chance of getting many types of cancer.

• Help your muscles to contract efficiently, affecting your overall metabolism.

• Help you get multi-vitamins in every bite and improve your energy levels.

• Improve your feelings and your overall energy levels.

• Change the look of your skin.

• Make you the hottie you are destined to be.

All of these health-giving, life-improving properties come from the same foods.

You deserve the best in your life. Your choice, your Life in Synergy.

All of the life giving health that you need coupled with the fun balance of a cookie, a cocktail or a slice of pizza.

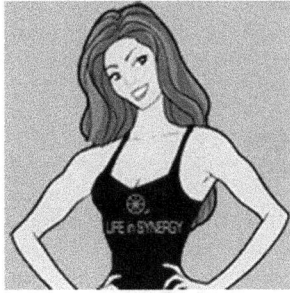

CHAPTER **14**

SELF-ASSESSMENT

Your journey to your greatest discovery begins now.

The journey to discover the you that lives each day at peace with your body, your weight and your choices.

I am selfish in my pursuit of your happiness and peace, to free each one of you from the treadmill of endless diets and emotions. When you emerge happy and more at peace with yourself, you bring peace and happiness to my world, as well. With your new way of life, you will have more free time to share with us all of your amazing talents, gifts and joy.

Creating your own Life in Synergy will spark those around you and will be a ripple effect of change. All of this is possible, just by taking time for the most important person in your life—you! There is a lifetime of information in this book; take your time, go back and review each section. Each time you reread a section, you will gain new insights and new discoveries about yourself.

This is the key to maintaining an interest in you. Remember, there is no absolute right or wrong. The ultimate goal is to feel great, love your body, do the physical activities that you enjoy, and properly care for your gift of life.

Learning about you

Your Life in Synergy: Understand and embrace the power of your brain.

The ultimate you: Stop managing and learn how to live.

Recognize your most important relationship: You will spend every moment of every day for the rest of your life with the most important person in your world, you. Realize that your relationship with yourself is the most important one in your world. Learn to love who you are.

Flip your pyramid: Life is impossible to balance if the entire world is pressing down on you, with everyone pulling you in a different direction all of the time. By learning your place at the top of your pyramid of self, you are not only properly supported by those in your life but you are better able to care for yourself and others.

Assess your current house of being: Step back and see where you are living now, the address and the area of your house of being that you occupy most often. Are you living in your body's attic, living room or garage?

Occupy your whole being not just one section: Are you a thinker, a decorator or a commuter? Utilize the exercises to learn to occupy your whole being, and spread out in your new amazing home. Explore all aspects of you.

Choose your new ideal house: Utilize the formula to figure out your number and eat your number every single day. You are using your brain, the world's strongest super computer, to program your ideal. The more consistent you are, the faster your brain will learn your preference, and the faster you will move into your dream home.

Learn about all of your food groups, including the chemicals: Awareness is key. The more you know the more you grow. Learn to bring the beige group and the toppers into balance.

Gender Matters: Men and women live by a different set of rules (which also accounts for our shoes being much cuter). Understand the food intake difference and learn to put yourself first in your life.

Choose foods that your brain recognizes: The easier it is for your brain to recognize the foods you are eating, the easier it is for your subconscious brain to self-regulate. Pick foods in their original package for a thinking-free day. The more plastic wrap, the more you have to analyze nutrition facts.

Understanding the role of exercise: Do not beat yourself up physically. Choose exercise and movement that you love. Be active throughout your day to increase your natural anti-inflammatories and fuel your brain.

Eat for Peace: "Will eating this today bring me peace today and tomorrow?" Break the addiction to disliking yourself. Waking up tomorrow in love with yourself and your body is the best comfort food of all.

Taste Bud Alignment: Assess your current utilization of each of your taste buds. Identify which ones are over stimulated, and explore the tastes that you are avoiding.

Do not forget to work out your insides: Eat sources of insoluble fiber to train your inside muscles, and eat soluble fiber for a daily detox and cleansing.

Feed all of your bodies: Recognize that your mental and emotional bodies need fueling and caring, as well. Before you reach for inflammatory foods, take the time to realize which part of you is really hungry or just tired. Do not put your physical body at risk.

Stop and assess before you eat: Who you are really feeding, and is there another source of fuel available? Before you reach for the cupcake, try indulging by singing your favorite song, reading a trashy novel or watching reality TV.

Be aware: Read your labels, and be informed about your vitamins and electrolytes.

You are complex and priceless.

Treat yourself accordingly.

Leaving judgement aside

Whew, that is a lot of information. Don't worry or judge yourself by what you do not know or by what you think are your shortcomings.

Remember, I have already given you an A. There is no room for judgment in a Life in Synergy. I have complete confidence in your success. You have all of the time in your world to learn about you. When we judge ourselves, we stop our learning cold in its tracks. There is a distinct difference between honest assessment and judgment; one helps you to see what areas you need to learn, and the other sends up a huge wall that prevents your forward progress on the road to your own Life in Synergy.

Go through each section and make a to do list of learning about you.

Showing interest

You and your body are two of the most interesting topics in the world. What a miracle the human body is. I always find it fascinating to see how much people learn about themselves once they have an injury or an illness. Being informed when you are sick or injured helps you to make better decisions about yourself and your care, but why wait for the negative? Spend just a few minutes per day learning about you, learning about how your body works, learning to communicate with your body instead of arguing with it.

Be the person in your group that changes the conversation to a positive instead of a negative. When you show interest in you, others around you will follow.

One of my favorite client stories is about Martha, a scientist. She works full-time in a local lab, and she is smart, funny and engaging. When I first met her and started talking with her about her life, she told me the most amazing thing. When she was in the 5th grade, her family doctor told her that she would always be fat. That it was her fate. Twenty years later, she walked into my studio and so that I could tell her that was absolutely not the case.

A light bulb went off in her head when I explained that her mass is a scientific determination of the number of calories needed to sustain a certain mass.

This is science. The judgment placed on her all those years ago was lifted, as well as her belief that her weight was a foregone conclusion. You can guess the rest of the story.

She started eating her number, learning about her muscles and communicating with her body instead of beating it up. Her posture changed, and her constant smile lights up a room. She was so excited to come in one day and tell me that she had become an inspiration for a coworker.

She is a living embodiment of a Life in Synergy. Each day, she learns more about herself and, without even trying, she inspires those around her to do the same. Talk about awesome.

Your story continues

Now it is time for you to recognize and realize your own Life in Synergy.

You are not alone on this journey. I am here cheering you on and supporting you in every step. Share your successes; inspire yourself and others by putting yourself first and living your own Life in Synergy. I send you all of my love and encouragement.

Love,

Helena

BIBLIOGRAPHY

Bray, GA Smith, SR et al. "Effect of dietary protein content on weight gain, energy expenditure, and body composition during overeating: a randomized controlled trial" Journal of the American Medical Association 307(1):47-55.

Fullerton-Smith, Jill & Oz, Mehmet C. The Truth About Food: What You Eat Can Change Your Life. New York Bloomsbury, 2007.

King, John E. The Mayo Clinic on Digestive Health. 2nd Ed. Baltimore Mayo Clinic, 2004.

Kurlansky, Mark. Salt: A World History New York Walker Publishing Company, 2001.

"Caloric Intake" About the Heart Maryland Heart Center, University of Maryland Medical Center Baltimore April, 2011.

McGee, Harold. On Food and Cooking: The Science and Lore of the Kitchen. Rev. Upd Ed. New York Scribner, 2004.

Yang, Qing "Gain weight by going diet?' Artificial sweeteners and the neurobiology of sugar cravings" Yale Journal of Biology and Medicine 83.2 2010: 101–108.

Do you want to know more about how to live your Life in Synergy?

•Check out the latest updates from from Helena!

•Find out why Helena LOVES Walking and Water®!

•Learn how to change your life by getting your Mind in Synergy!

•Follow Life in Synergy on Facebook and Twitter!

www.lifeinsynergy.com

www.facebook.com/LifeInSynergy

www.twitter.com/LifeInSynergy

Want a FREE digital download of the Nutritional Alignment® Recipe Book?
Just send your purchase receipt to - team@lifeinsynergy.com and we will send you your FREE Nutritional Alignment® Recipe Book!!

Please spread good Karma!

Send us a review on Amazon,
We would truly appreciate it!

:)

www.ingramcontent.com/pod-product-compliance
Lightning Source LLC
Chambersburg PA
CBHW050352280326
41933CB00010BA/1434